W0043416

Clinician's Manual on Lupus

Clinician's Manual on Lupus

Editor
Professor Graham R V Hughes MD FRCP
Head of The London Lupus Centre,
London Bridge Hospital

Dr Shirish Sangle MD
Associate Consultant, Lupus Unit,
St Thomas' Hospital, London

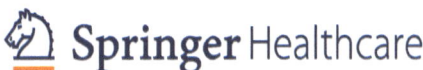 Springer Healthcare

Published by Springer Healthcare Ltd, 236 Gray's Inn Road, London, WC1X 8HB, UK.

www.springerhealthcare.com

© 2012 Springer Healthcare, a part of Springer Science+Business Media.

British Library Cataloguing-in-Publication Data.

A catalogue record for this book is available from the British Library.

ISBN 978-1-908517-48-7

Commissioning editor: Dinah Alam
Project editor: Katrina Dorn
Designer: Joe Harvey
Artworker: Sissan Mollerfors
Production: Marina Maher

Contents

Author biographies   ix

PART ONE   The growth of lupus

1   Lupus: An introduction   **1**
Distribution of lupus   1
Is lupus on the increase?   2
What has changed in lupus?   2

2   What is lupus?   **5**
Who gets lupus?   6
Clinical features   7

PART TWO   Lupus organ by organ

3   Skin   **11**
Livedo reticularis   13
Subacute cutaneous lupus erythematosus   13
Discoid lupus   15
Lupus profundus   16
Alopecia   16

4   Tendons and joints   **19**
Tendons   19
Joints   19
Muscles   21

5   Kidney   **23**
Pathology   23
Clinical features   24
Vascular lesions   25
Treatment   25

6   The brain   **27**
Mechanisms   27

Stroke   28

Headache   29

Memory loss   29

Seizures   29

Myelopathy   30

Neuropsychiatric features   30

Peripheral neuropathy   30

Treatment   31

7 Heart and blood vessels   33

Heart   33

Atheroma   35

Vasculitis   36

8 Liver and gastrointestinal tract 39

Liver   39

Gastrointestinal tract   39

9 Blood   41

White blood cells   42

Red cells   42

Platelets   42

PART THREE   Diagnosis and treatment

10 Diagnosing lupus   45

Clinical clues   46

Diagnostic criteria   46

Laboratory tests   48

Antiphospholipid antibodies   50

Full blood count   51

Complement levels   51

C-reactive protein   51

Urinalysis and electrolytes   51

Other investigations   52

11 Treatment   **53**

General management   53

Drug therapy   54

PART FOUR   Lupus-like disorders

12 Sjögren's syndrome   **63**

Pathology   64

Clinical features   65

Eye   66

Mouth and gastrointestinal tract   66

Vagina and bladder   67

Kidney   67

Nervous system   67

Blood   67

Purpura   68

Other autoimmune diseases   68

Malignancy   69

Diagnosis   69

Schirmer's tear test   69

Immunology   70

Other diagnostic tests   71

Etiology   72

Treatment   72

13 Hughes syndrome
    (the antiphospholipid syndrome)   **73**

Introduction   74

Blood   74

Pregnancy   74

Brain   76

Heart   76

Other organs   76

Treatment   79

The future   80

14 Mixed connective tissue disease (and overlap syndromes)   81

Clinical features   81

Immunology   83

Outcome   83

15 Vasculitis   85

Classification   85

Wegener's granulomatosis   85

Polyarteritis nodosa   91

Takayasu's arteritis   92

PART FIVE   Lupus-related topics

16 Lupus-related topics   97

Lupus and pregnancy   97

Lupus in children   97

Lupus and late arterial disease   98

Lupus and malignancy   98

Drug-induced lupus   99

Lupus: soil versus seed   100

Author biographies

Professor Graham Hughes is often referred to as "the father of lupus" in the UK. Trained at the London Hospital, he went on to spend two years in New York under the leadership of Dr Charles Christian, where he worked on the introduction of the DNA-binding test.

In 1971, he opened the lupus clinic at Hammersmith Hospital before moving to St Thomas' Hospital where he set up the Louise Coote Lupus Unit, a specialist unit dealing uniquely with lupus and related diseases. In 1983, he described the antiphospholipid syndrome, now known as Hughes Syndrome, and in 1991 was awarded the International League of Associations for Rheumatology (ILAR) prize for this work. He also instituted an annual postgraduate meeting "Ten Topics in Rheumatology", now in its 25th year, with satellite "Ten Topics" meetings in six countries.

Professor Hughes is founder and editor of the international journal *LUPUS*.

Other honors include Master of the American College of Rheumatology and doctor honoris causa degrees from the University of Marseille and University of Barcelona.

Professor Hughes is best known for his work with patients and is Life President of the patients' charity Lupus UK.

Shirish Sangle is an associate consultant at the Louise Coote Lupus Unit, St Thomas' Hospital, London. He has been working with Professor Hughes since 2000. His main fields of research include livedo reticularis, non-traumatic bone fractures, and arterial stenosis in Hughes syndrome.

PART ONE

The growth of lupus

Chapter 1

Lupus: An introduction

Forty years ago lupus (systemic lupus erythematosus) was widely regarded as a rare, largely untreatable disease: at best, requiring high dose steroids; at worst, ending in renal failure. However, lupus is now recognized as an important and relatively common disease affecting up to 1 in 800 women; it is more common than multiple sclerosis or leukemia. In many countries, lupus is now seen by every primary care practitioner. It is very treatable, and most patients diagnosed early can expect a normal lifespan. It is predominantly a disease of young women (most commonly affecting women between the ages of 15–45) but can affect men as well. Pregnancy, once contraindicated in lupus, is now largely successful.

Distribution of lupus

Possibly due to the photosensitivity seen in many patients, lupus is more common in sunny countries. For example, there are higher rates of lupus in Spain and Italy than in England or Scotland.

In some countries in East Asia — notably Singapore, the Philippines, Indonesia and China — lupus appears particularly common, overtaking rheumatoid arthritis in prevalence (Figure 1.1).

There are also ethnic differences, with lupus being more common (and more severe) in Asian and African patients than in Northern Europeans. Lupus is especially common in the African-American and Afro-Caribbean communities, although strangely, it is considered rare in Africa itself.

Global distribution of lupus

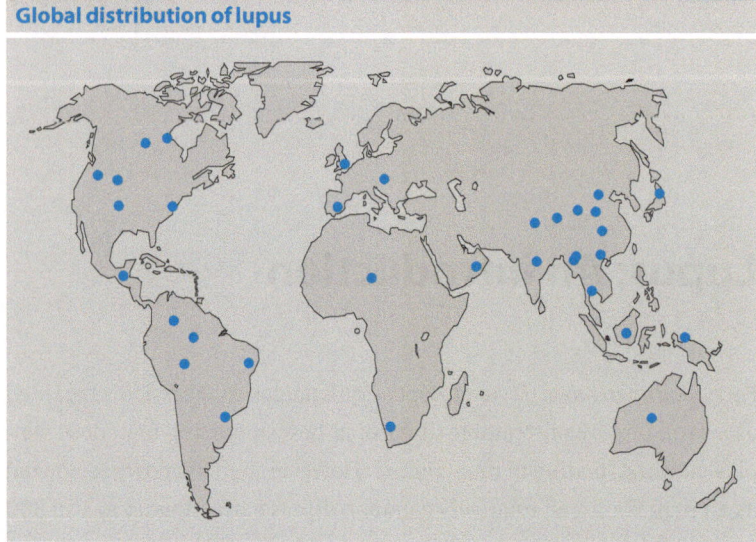

Figure 1.1 Global distribution of lupus. Global incidence of lupus is estimated to be between 1 to 10 cases per 100,000. Prevalence is highest among Asian, African-American, Afro-Caribbean and Hispanic-American populations. Dots indicate areas of higher incidence of lupus.

Is lupus on the increase?

Yes, very much so. One of the questions commonly asked is if lupus is becoming more common. It is certainly true that disease rates can fluctuate; for instance, in the UK, rheumatoid arthritis appears to be waning. The likely answer is that with greater awareness, many more cases of lupus are now being diagnosed.

Another theory for the possible rise in lupus is the 'hygiene theory.' Today infants and children are exposed to far fewer infections and those who develop infections are treated with antibiotics. Thus the immune system does not fully develop protective infection-fighting immune responses.

What has changed in lupus?

Recently, there have been major changes in understanding and managing lupus. One of the most important changes has been increased awareness. Lupus was once relegated to the 'rare diseases' section of medical textbooks. Doctors received little in the way of exposure to or education about lupus and the general public were largely unaware of it. Today, media pieces on lupus regularly appear in magazines and on the internet, radio and television. A number of cases of lupus in well-known showbusiness personalities have also raised its profile. And most importantly, patients' self-help groups have sprung up all over the world, providing patients with information about their diagnosis and disease management advice.

As a result of increased awareness and testing advances, earlier diagnosis is now possible using extremely sensitive tests, such as double stranded DNA (dsDNA)-antibody testing, reducing the time to diagnosis and treatment in a large proportion of patients. Finally, more effective treatments are now available, allowing patients to live longer, healthier lives. These treatments will be discussed in detail in Chapter 11.

Chapter 2

What is lupus?

Lupus is a condition in which the immune system, for some currently unexplained reason, becomes overactive. In lupus, the body produces antibodies (which can appear years before the disease itself; Figure 2.1) and these in turn can damage sensitive organs and tissues, notably the small blood vessels (vasculitis; Figure 2.2) and the kidney.

Other functions of the immune system can also become faulty, including immune protection (T cell function) and apoptosis, the removal of tissue waste from cell breakdown (Figure 2.3).

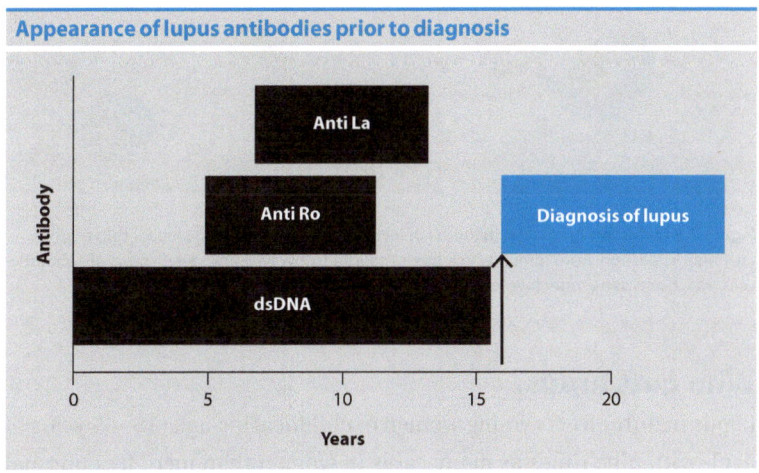

Appearance of lupus antibodies prior to diagnosis

Figure 2.1 Appearance of lupus antibodies prior to diagnosis. Lupus antibodies (eg, extractable nuclear antigen [ENA], double-stranded DNA [dsDNA], anti-La, anti-Ro) can appear up to 15 years before the clinical manifestation of lupus.

Vasculitis

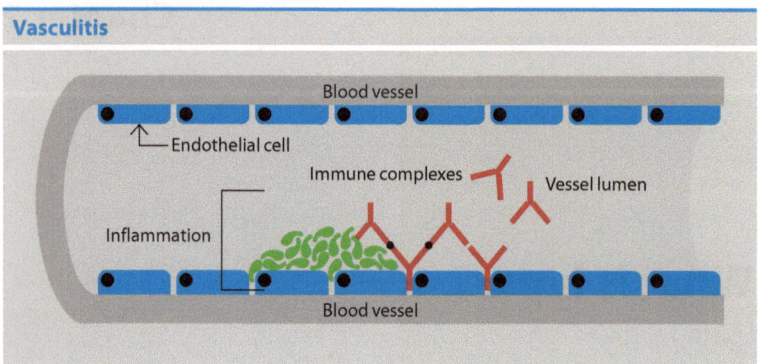

Figure 2.2 Vasculitis. Vasculitis occurs when immune complexes deposited in the blood vessels lead to inflammation.

Defective apoptosis in lupus

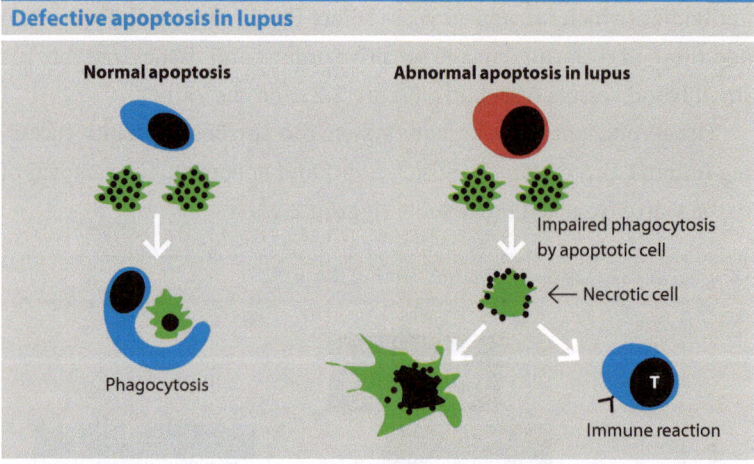

Figure 2.3 Defective apoptosis in lupus. Defective disposal of apoptotic (dead) cells triggers an immune reaction. Autoimmunity in lupus is thought to involve improper disposal of apoptotic cells, which acts as a trigger for the production of characteristic auto-antibodies.

Who gets lupus?

Lupus mainly affects young women of childbearing age (15–45 years of age), with nine times as many cases in women than men. It is unusual for new cases of lupus to develop after menopause. Lupus can sometimes run in families, especially when other autoimmune conditions such as thyroid disease, rheumatoid arthritis, or Hughes syndrome are prominent (Figure 2.4).

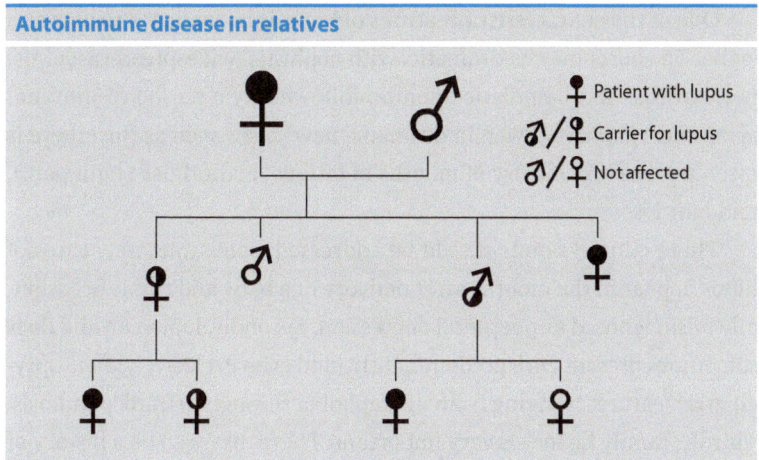

Autoimmune disease in relatives

Patient with lupus
Carrier for lupus
Not affected

Figure 2.4 Autoimmune disease in relatives. While there is a genetic basis for the development of lupus, it is often triggered by a mixture of environmental and genetic factors. There is an increased concordance in identical twins and non-identical siblings.

Clinical features

Common early symptoms are non specific and include fatigue, flu-like features such as aches and pains, and low-grade fever. There may be hair loss, skin rashes and chest discomfort from pleurisy. The hands may show digital blisters and Raynaud's phenomenon. Urine testing may show proteinuria.

Sometimes, however, the onset may be more dramatic, with pericarditis, widespread 'pain all over', or neurological features including headaches and seizures.

A common presenting scenario is of a woman between 20 and 30 years of age with ongoing fatigue, faint skin rashes (commonly on the V-neck, eyebrows and cheeks), aches and pains but no joint swelling, and some hair loss. There may have been a past history of headaches or migraine, growing pains, or a prolonged episode of glandular fever.

Because lupus can have a rather slow onset, diagnosis can sometimes be delayed. Fortunately, the main blood test for lupus (anti-dsDNA antibody) is very specific for the disease. Indeed it is now known that positive antibody tests (such as an anti-dsDNA) may antedate clinical diagnosis by months or even years.

One of the characteristic features of lupus is its tendency to wax and wane. The onset may be dramatic, with nephritis, widespread vasculitis, pericarditis, and hemolytic anemia, followed by a period of minimal symptoms. However, even in dramatic 'new' cases such as this, there is often a preceding history of months of fatigue, arthralgias (joint pain), and hair loss.

Three clinical points should be addressed: sometimes new cases of lupus appear in the months after delivery of a baby and this is occasionally misdiagnosed as puerperal depression. Secondly, lupus can and does sometimes present with predominantly (and even exclusively) neuropsychiatric features, ranging from agoraphobia through to frank psychosis. Thirdly, family history is very important. There may well be a history of other autoimmune diseases, including lupus, in other family members.

PART TWO

Lupus organ by organ

Chapter 3

Skin

A variety of skin rashes is seen in lupus. The most well known is the classical 'butterfly' rash on the cheeks and the bridge of the nose (Figure 3.1). However, this rash is seen in less than half of all patients.

The most common rash is a widespread flat pink rash, that is prominent on the V-neck, face (including eyebrows), hands, and lower limbs (Figure 3.2).

These rashes are often sun-provoked, coming on after a holiday, for example (Figure 3.3). It should be noted, however, that sun-sensitivity is not a universal feature.

Butterfly rash in lupus

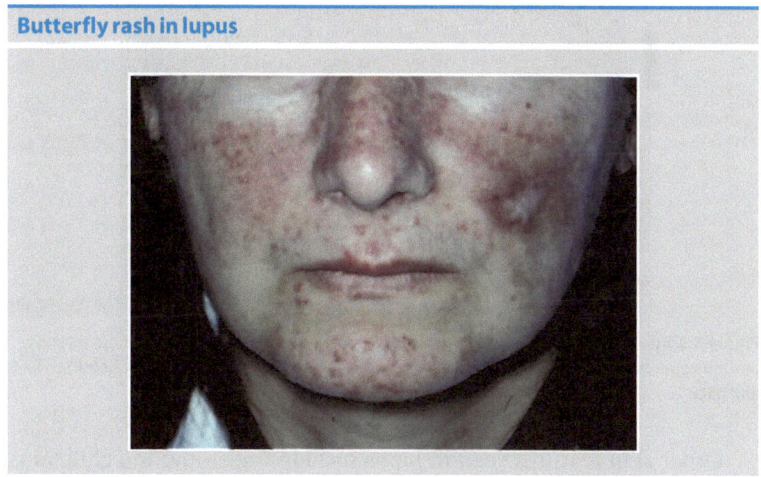

Figure 3.1 Butterfly rash in lupus. A classic malar 'butterfly rash' affecting the cheeks and nose. Patient also has scarring on the left cheek, suggesting additional discoid lesion.

Flat pink rash on neck and arms

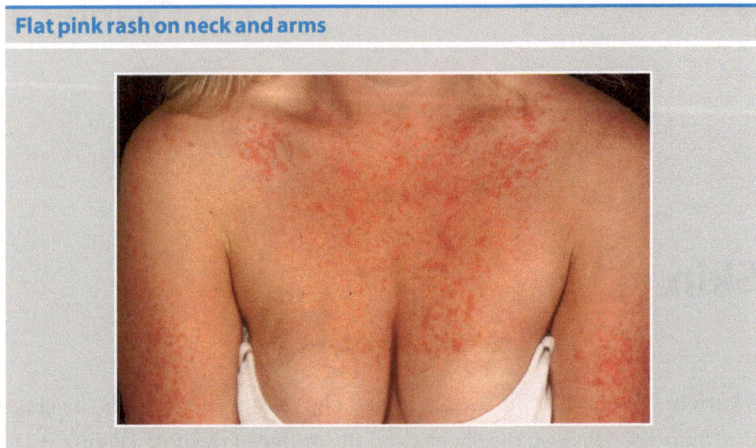

Figure 3.2 Flat pink rash on neck and arms. The most common rash associated with lupus, typically distributed across the face, arms, hands, and V-neck area of the anterior chest.

Sun-provoked rash on back

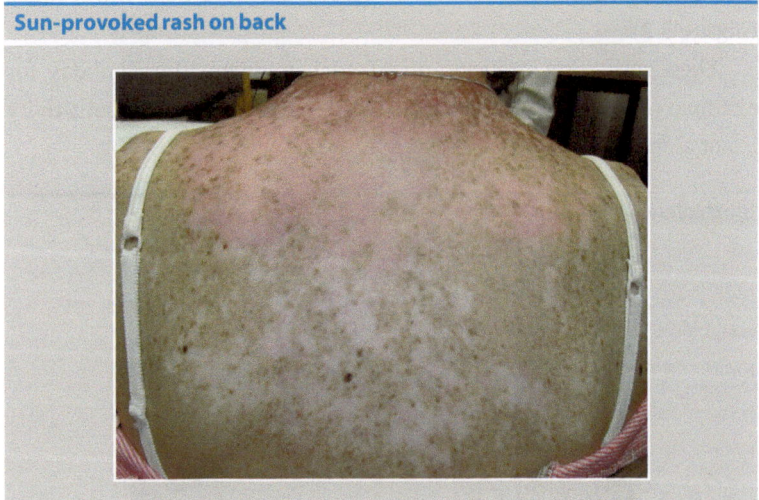

Figure 3.3 Sun-provoked rash on back. Rashes associated with lupus are often photosensitive and are aggravated by sun exposure. These rashes tend to appear on the face, arms, hands, chest, and back.

Other skin features seen in lupus include finger and toe chilblains (Figure 3.4; more common in children), subungual splinter hemorrhages, mouth ulcers, and cutaneous vasculitis (lesions commonly seen on the elbows and tips of fingers and toes).

Hand chilblains

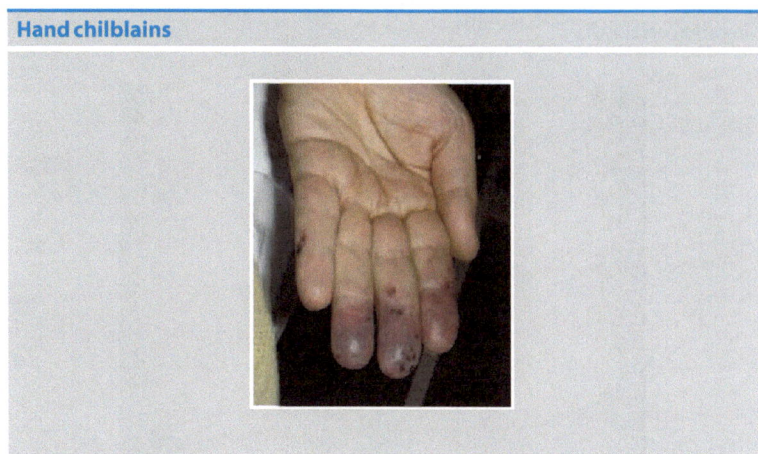

Figure 3.4 Hand chilblains. Discoloration caused by chilblains, a type of vasculitis triggered by exposure to cold temperatures. It can also be exacerbated by smoking.

A number of skin-related features deserve separate comment:

- Livedo reticularis
- Subacute cutaneous lupus erythematosus (SCLE)
- Discoid lupus
- Lupus profundus
- Alopecia

Livedo reticularis

A peculiar lattice-like condition (known by some patients as 'corned beef skin'; Figure 3.5) is seen in a number of conditions including vasculitis and cryoglobulinemia. It is seen in lupus, but is especially prominent in patients with Hughes syndrome (see Chapter 13). It is a particularly important symptom because of its association with increased risk of headache and stroke.

Subacute cutaneous lupus erythematosus

Subacute cutaneous lupus erythematosus (SCLE) is an easily recognized skin lesion, often circular or doughnut shaped, that develops especially on the upper chest (Figure 3.6) and is sometimes mistaken for a fungal lesion. It is clinically associated with anti-Ro/La antibodies. SCLE is often very

Livedo reticularis

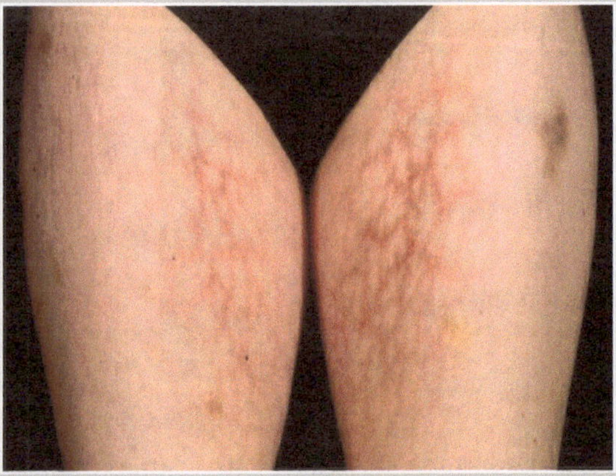

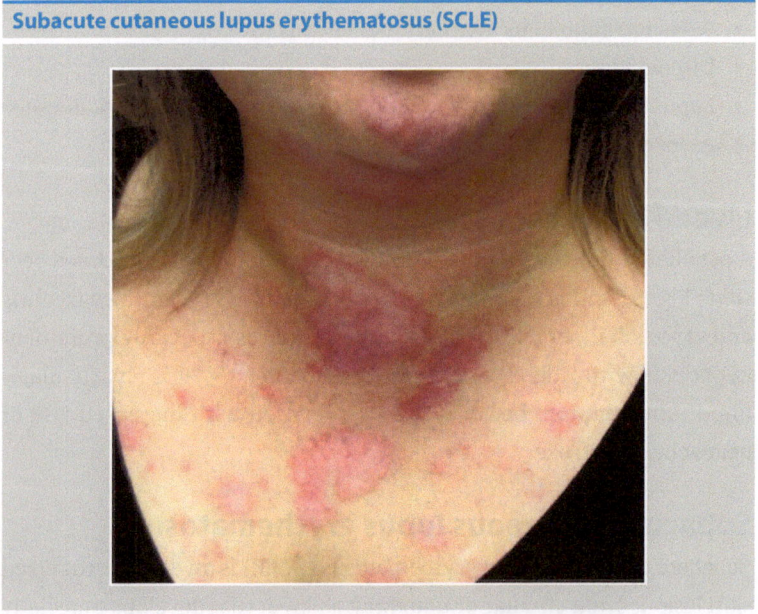

Figure 3.5 Livedo reticularis. A lattice-like discoloration of the skin ('corned beef skin') caused by poor circulation. Livedo reticularis is found in patients with lupus, but is more often seen in Hughes syndrome and vasculitis.

Subacute cutaneous lupus erythematosus (SCLE)

Figure 3.6 Subacute cutaneous lupus erythematosus (SCLE). Well defined erythematous discoid skin lesions shown on the chest and neck are typical of SCLE. This non-scarring rash is linked to photosensitivity and is associated with anti-Ro and anti-La antibodies.

photosensitive, is occasionally associated with Sjögren's syndrome (see Chapter 12) and tends to have a good prognosis. In pregnancy, maternal anti-Ro antibodies can cross to the intrauterine fetus, leading to a similar rash in the newborn (neonatal lupus) which is usually benign. Less benign is the association of anti-Ro antibodies with rare infant congenital heart block (see Chapter 16).

Discoid lupus

Although discoid lupus generally has a better prognosis than systemic lupus erythematosus, it can nevertheless be widespread and disfiguring. Discoid lupus causes skin to become scaly, patchy, and raised and commonly affects the scalp (Figure 3.7), the face, and the limbs (often in small patches resembling psoriasis). Blood tests for systemic lupus are usually negative/normal for lupus antibodies and most patients (although not all) respond well to antimalarial treatment.

Discoid lupus lesions on the scalp

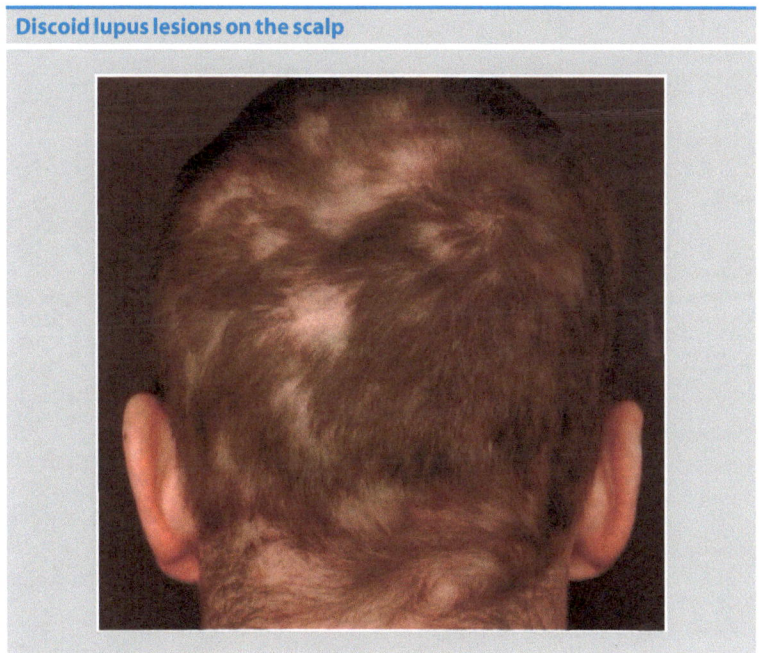

Figure 3.7 Discoid lupus lesions on the scalp. Discoid lupus affecting the scalp may cause hair loss due to permanent scarring. Distribution can be anywhere on the skin, but it is most commonly seen on areas of the body exposed to the sun (eg, cheeks, ears, and scalp).

Lupus profundus

Rarely, patients with lupus can develop a lumpy deep subcutaneous panniculitis. This condition often presents with numerous, slightly tender subcutaneous lumps, with puckering of the overlying skin. Lesions commonly affect the limbs and trunk, but occasionally cause disfiguring lesions on the face.

Alopecia

Hair loss is a common and important feature of lupus and is an early indication of a flare of the disease. Occasionally, it can be acute and severe. Fortunately, in almost all cases, total regrowth of the hair occurs once the disease is brought under control. The occasional exception is the patient with discoid lupus where inadequately treated disease can lead to permanent (and usually patchy) scalp scaring and baldness (Figure 3.8).

Alopecia in lupus

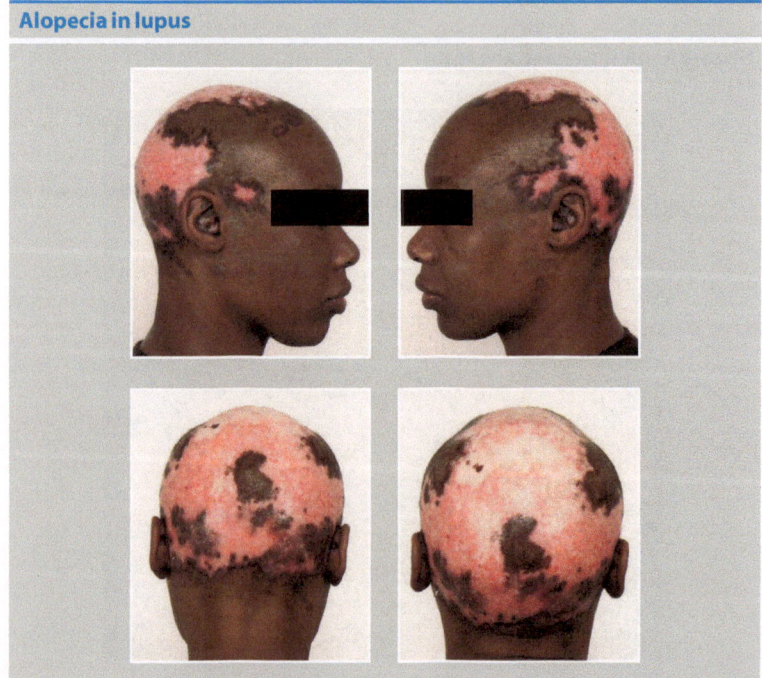

Figure 3.8 Alopecia in lupus. Alopecia and sever scarring in discold lupus.

Diagnosis of cutaneous lupus is generally straightforward, given the background history and findings. In the past, skin biopsy with histology was widely used. Immunofluoresence of the biopsy characteristically showed a band of immunofluorescence (immune complexes and complement) at the dermo-epidermal junction (Figure 3.9), and was called the 'lupus band test'. However, this test is now rarely used as other non-invasive tests are available.

Lupus immunofluorescence band test on skin biopsy

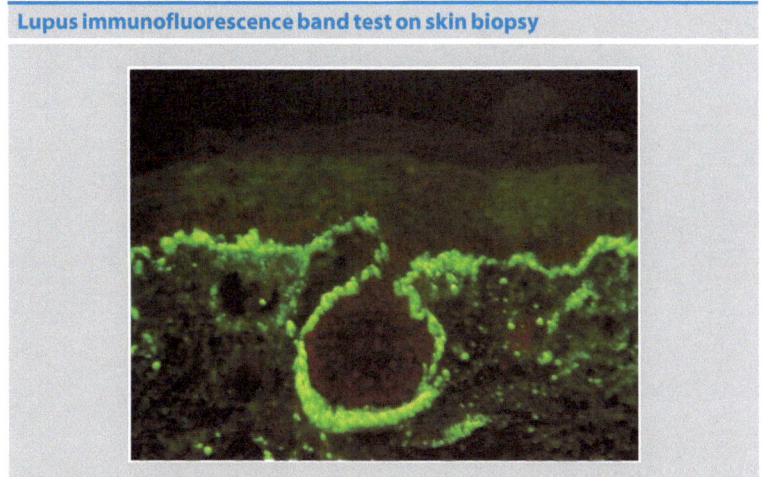

Figure 3.9 Lupus immunofluorescence band test on skin biopsy. An immunofluorescence staining to identify a band of immune complexes and complement at the dermo-epidermal junction.

Chapter 4

Tendons and joints

Possibly the most common symptom in lupus is aches and pains. These can be severe, often with 'pain all over'. The symptoms fluctuate and with clinical remission can disappear completely. Unlike rheumatoid arthritis, chronic joint swelling is rare and joint erosion is very unusual. The symptom of widespread pain can result from a mix of muscle, joint and tendon inflammation.

Tendons

Tendon involvement is an important feature of lupus. Patients often complain of stiffness in the fingers, with difficulty in straightening the fingers fully. There may be tendon crepitus or even triggering. Occasionally, larger tendons such as the Achilles may be involved and tendon rupture is an occasional complication.

An extreme (although unusual) manifestation of tendon involvement in lupus is the development of severe deformities in the fingers (and sometimes the toes) due to ongoing tendon contractures, a condition known as Jaccoud's arthritis (Figure 4.1A and B).

Joints

While the joints themselves largely escape erosive damage in lupus, one major problem in some patients is avascular necrosis, or cellular bone death, usually as a result of high dosage steroids and most commonly leading to necrosis of the head of the femur.

Jaccoud's arthopathy

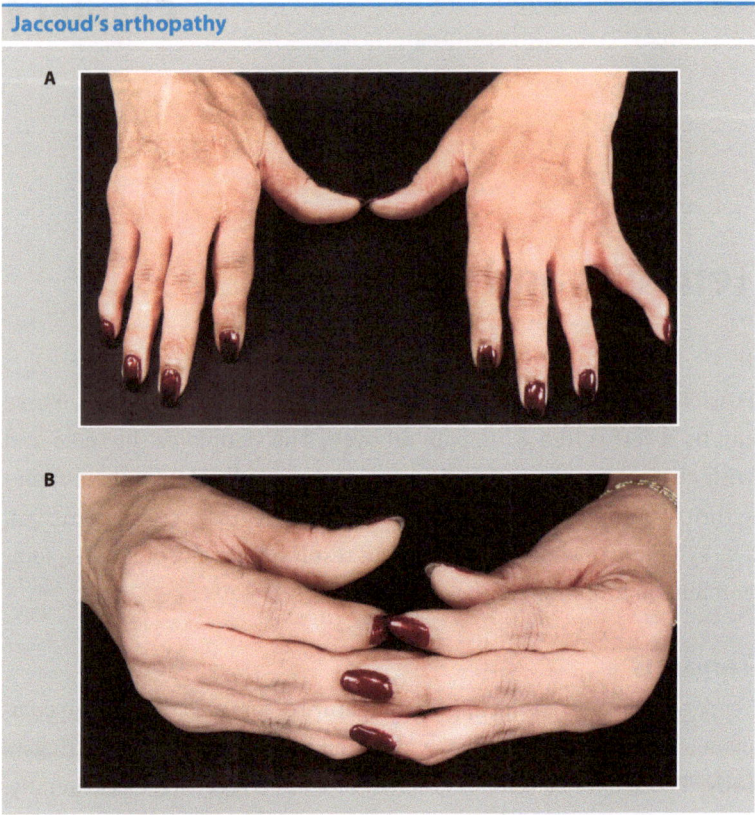

Figure 4.1 A and B Jaccoud's arthopathy. Hand showing deformity caused by Jaccoud's arthopathy. It is characterized by non-erosive joint deformation and is thought to be caused by tendon inflammation and contracture.

The earliest signs of avascular necrosis of the femur head are groin discomfort and limitation of hip rotation. MRI may show characteristic changes (Figure 4.2A) long before X-ray changes appear (Figure 4.2B). Management of early avascular necrosis generally requires avoidance of weight-bearing. Occasionally, surgical decompression is helpful. Ultimately, total hip replacement is the treatment of choice.

While active widespread synovitis is unusual in lupus, it is less unusual in mixed connective tissue disease (MCTD; see Chapter 14). Some MCTD patients suffer troublesome symmetric small joint pain and swelling often resembling early rheumatoid arthritis.

MRI showing avascular necrosis of the hip

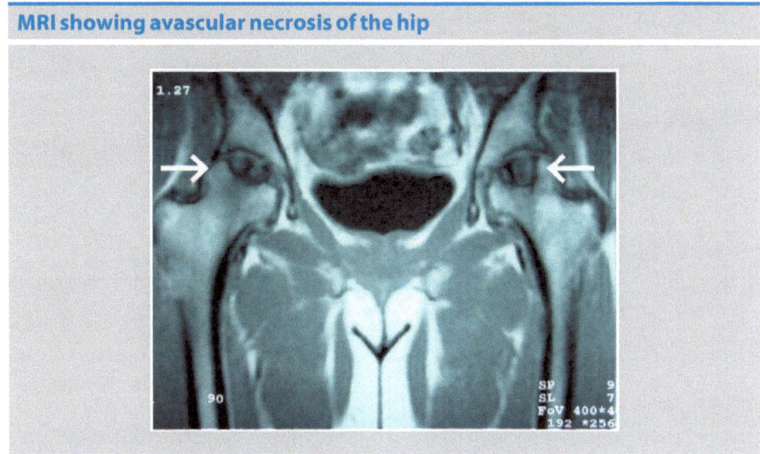

Figure 4.2A MRI showing avascular necrosis of both hip joints.

X-ray showing avascular necrosis of hip

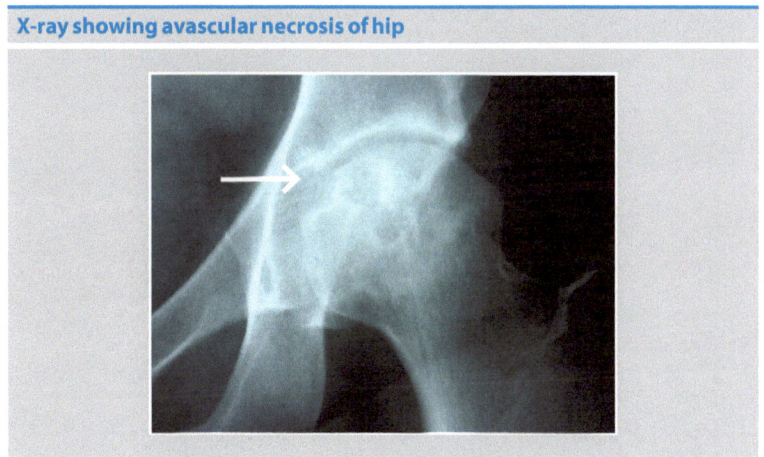

Figure 4.2B **X-ray showing avascular necrosis of the hip.** Avascular necrosis of the hip is also observed in lupus patients, especially those receiving corticosteroids. Arrow shows area of necrosis of the head of the femur.

Muscles

While aches and pains are a feature of lupus, true inflammatory myositis is rare. (Raised muscle enzymes are sometimes seen in patients on statins). On the contrary, in MCTD, myositis can be troublesome and on occasion severe, requiring combinations of steroid and immunosuppressive treatments (particulary methotrexate).

Chapter 5

Kidney

One of the most feared complications of lupus is nephritis (inflammation in the kidney), which can develop insidiously and, in undiagnosed or untreated patients, may potentially lead to renal failure. However, with greater awareness and early treatment, the prognosis of lupus nephritis has improved markedly and the majority of cases can be brought into remission.

Pathology

The pathology of the glomerular injury in lupus is classified into six classes (in accordance with International Society of Nephrology [ISN] and Renal Pathology Society [RPS]).

Class I	Minimal glomerular disease (Figure 5.1A).
Class II	Mesangial proliferative lupus nephritis (Figure 5.1B).
Class III	Focal proliferative glomerulonephritis (Figure 5.1C).
Class IV	Diffuse segmental proliferative glomerulonephritis (necrosis, cellular crescents, variable sclerosis; Figure 5.1D).
Class V	Membranous (Figure 5.1E).
Class VI	Sclerosing nephropathy (fibrosis, hyalinised glomeruli, "tombstones") (Figure 5.1F).

Immunofluorescence may reveal deposits containing immunoglobulin.

Renal pathology of lupus nephritis (Class I-VI)

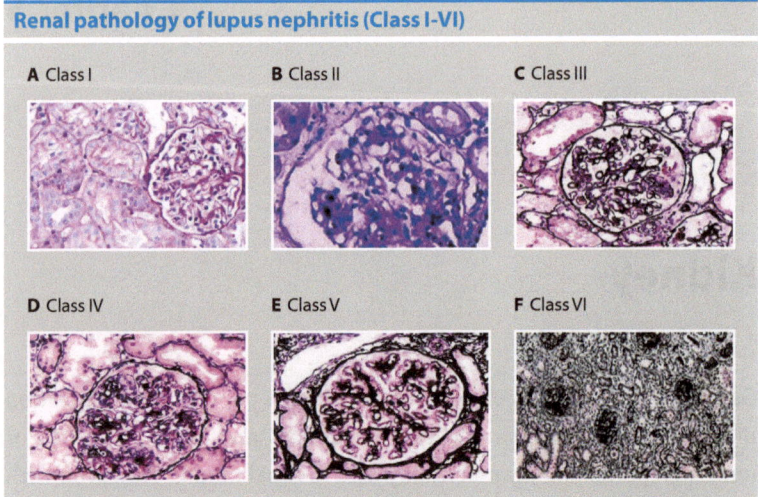

Figure 5.1A–F Renal pathology of lupus nephritis (Class I-VI). A, Class I: Minimal mesangial lupus nephritis (no treatment necessary); B, Class II: Mesangial proliferative lupus nephritis; C, Class III: Focal segmental glomerulonephritis (<50% glomeruli are affected); D, Class IV: Diffuse lupus nephritis (>50% of glomeruli are affected); E, Class V: Membranous lupus nephritis; F, Class VI: Advanced sclerosing lupus nephritis (beyond treatment with immunosuppressive therapy).

Because the histological picture is critical to the choice of treatment (for example, there is little point in prescribing strong immunosuppressives for a kidney with essentially 'dead' glomeruli), renal biopsy is widely considered vital in the early clinical assessment of a patient with lupus in whom proteinuria or other renal sequelae are present. Modern renal biopsy under radiological guidance with a fine needle is now regarded as very safe (though not sufficiently risk-free to be considered in a patient with a solitary kidney).

Clinical features

The most common early manifestation of nephritis is proteinuria; as such, it is our policy to teach patients with lupus to self-test the urine monthly in cases of suspected active nephritis. Regular urinalysis is a vital part of lupus assessment, checking for proteinuria and active urinary sediment or casts. More severe renal involvement can lead to nephrotic syndrome, hypertension, or even renal failure.

Vascular lesions

Patients with lupus who test positive for antiphospholipid (aPL) antibodies and those patients with primary antiphospholipid syndrome (APS or Hughes syndrome) are more prone to intraglomerular thrombosis (Figure 5.2), a feature which can add significantly to renal impairment if not treated. Thrombosis in larger vessels such as the renal artery and renal vein can also occur in Hughes syndrome. Interestingly, patients with Hughes syndrome can develop focal stenotic lesions in the renal artery, leading to hypertension.

Treatment

The use of drugs such as cyclophosphamide, azathioprine, rituximab, belimumab, and mycophenolate mofetil have vastly improved the outlook for renal lupus, with a move away from prolonged high-dose steroids. For those patients developing renal failure in lupus, dialysis and transplant are usually successful. In fact, it is unusual for lupus to flare after a renal transplant.

Renal pathology in Hughes syndrome: thrombotic microangiopathy

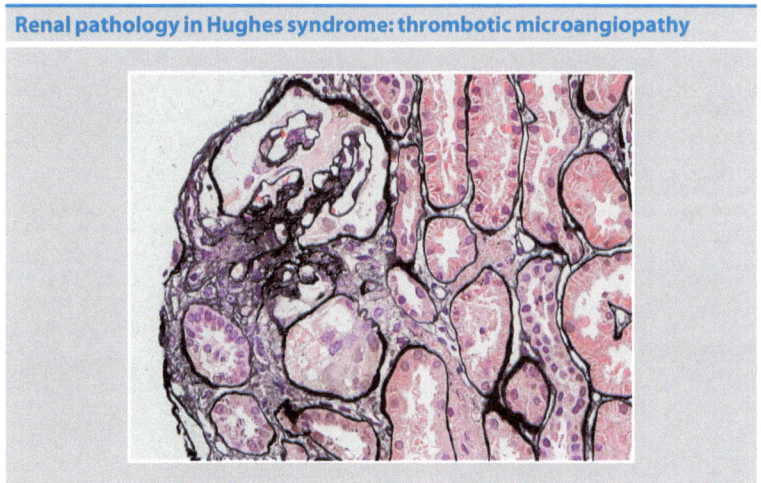

Figure 5.2 Renal pathology in Hughes syndrome: thrombotic microangiopathy. Micro-infarcts in the renal blood vessels. Thrombotic microangiopathy may lead to chronic renal impairment.

Chapter 6

The brain

Lupus has been described as "a predominantly neurological disease in which other organs may also be involved." However, the percentage of patients with lupus with neurological involvement varies, depending largely on definition and inclusion criteria. Nevertheless, it is now recognized that brain features of lupus are more common than previously thought, especially when more sensitive neurocognitive impairment is fully included.

Mechanisms

There are three main mechanisms by which brain dysfunction is thought to arise: direct antibody attack (a number of antineuronal antibodies are now recognized), inflammatory vasculitis, and thrombosis (Figure 6.1).

Until recently, most clinical neurological features in lupus were attributed to 'central nervous system vasculitis'. Not so today, as true inflammatory vasculitis is rare. Possibly the most important mechanism is cerebral blood flow impairment which can cause thrombosis and blood 'sludging', leading to ischemia (the latter is linked to Hughes syndrome; see Chapter 13).

Indeed the overlap between aPL-associated neurological features and lupus-associated neurological features is so great that a major rethink concerning the relative contributions of the two disorders is underway. This is not entirely academic as decisions regarding treatment, such as whether to prescribe anti-inflammatory corticosteroids versus anticoagulants, are dependent on widely differing etiologies.

Brain injury in lupus

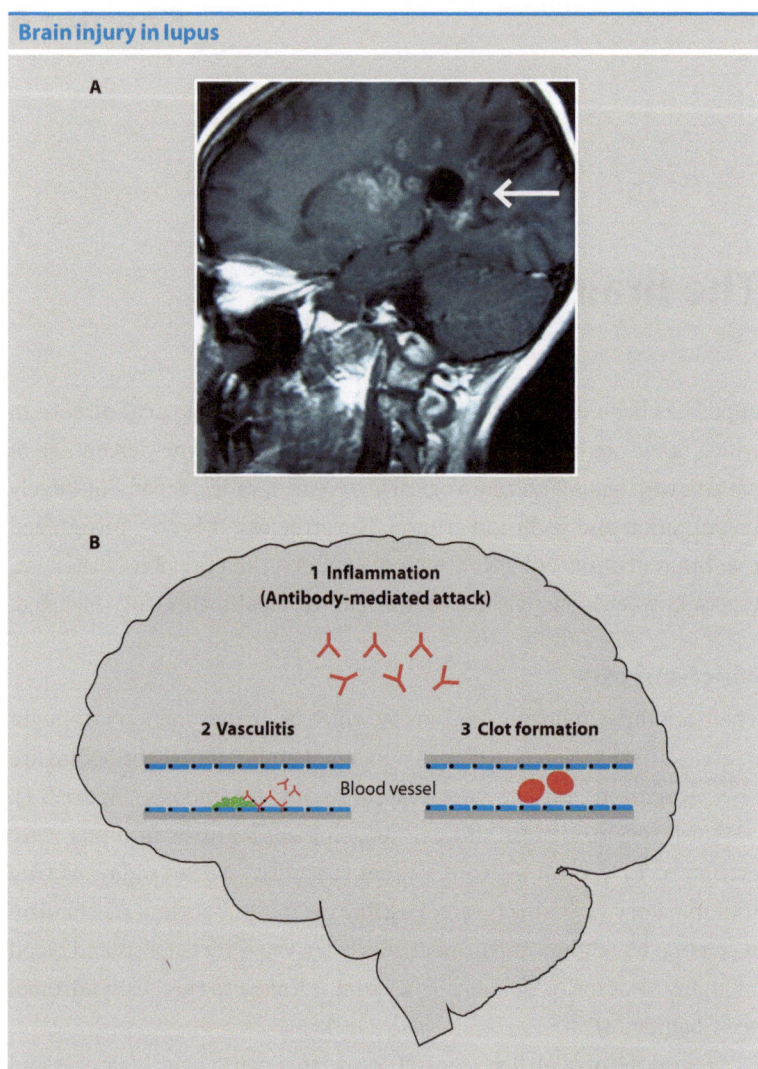

Figure 6.1A and B Brain injury in lupus. A, CT scan showing brain injury; B, Brain injury in lupus can be caused by: 1, Antibody - mediated attack; 2, Cerebral vasculitis; 3, Blood sludging and thrombosis (often seen in Hughes syndrome).

Stroke

One of the most feared complications of lupus is stroke. Stroke is strongly associated with aPL antibodies and Hughes syndrome. This topic is further discussed in Chapter 13 (Figure 6.2).

Major stroke in a patient with lupus

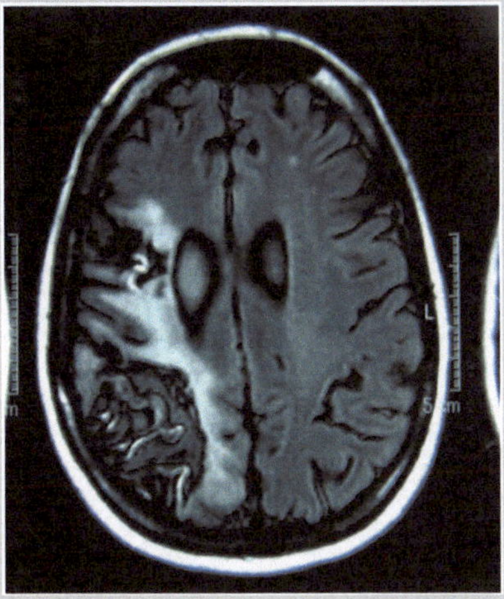

Figure 6.2 Major stroke in a patient with lupus. Brain CT scan image showing a major stroke. Patients with lupus are at greater risk of ischemic stroke due to higher likelihood of vasculitis, thrombosis, and Libman-Sacks endocarditis..

Headache

One of the most common features of lupus is headache, which is often frequent and migrainous. Sometimes patients with headache respond to steroids but more commonly react to anti-aggregants or anticoagulants. In patients with Hughes syndrome, headaches can be a precursor to transient ischemic attacks.

Memory loss

This can be mild and a nonspecific feature of chronic inflammatory illness. In Hughes syndrome, memory loss may be severe and give rise to fears of Alzheimer's disease.

Seizures

During the early, severe phase of lupus, seizures are not uncommon (Figure 6.3). As lupus responds to treatment, these become uncommon. Seizures (ranging from grand mal to temporal lobe epilepsy) are more common in patients that are aPL-positive (see Chapter 13).

Seizures in lupus

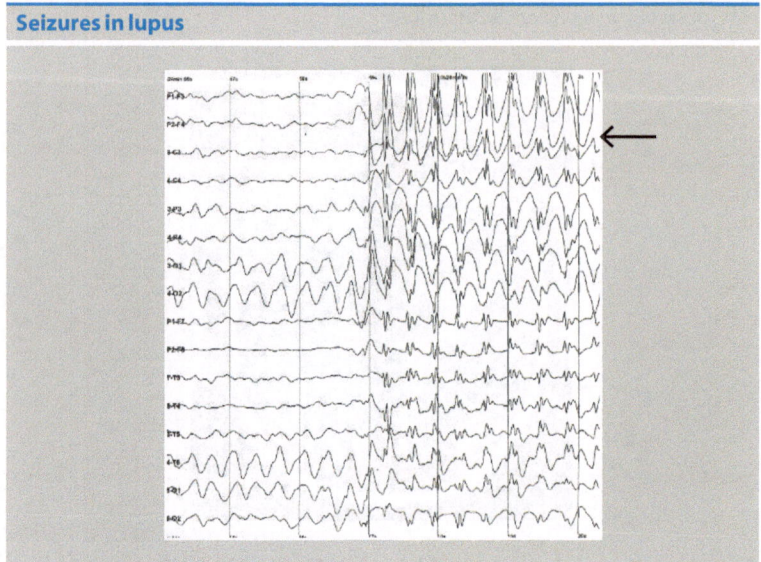

Figure 6.3 Seizures in lupus. Electroencephalograph (EEG) showing a seizure in a patient with lupus. Arrow shows abnormal wave pattern in a seizure.

Myelopathy

A rare but serious manifestation of lupus is transverse myelitis (Figure 6.4). Usually acute, it will respond to speedy treatment, which is typically a combination of steroids, immunosuppressives, and (increasingly) anticoagulants.

Neuropsychiatric features

Active lupus can lead to a wide range of neuropsychiatric manifestations. Depression is common, as are phobias. Psychosis can be a prominent presentation. Generally responsive to a combination of antipsychotic and lupus medication, lupus-related psychosis rarely leads to long-term neuropsychiatric sequelae.

Peripheral neuropathy

As distinct from vasculitis, peripheral neuropathy is uncommon in lupus. Other problems encountered in lupus include balance disorders, atypical multiple sclerosis, movement disorders, balance difficulties,

Transverse myelitis in lupus

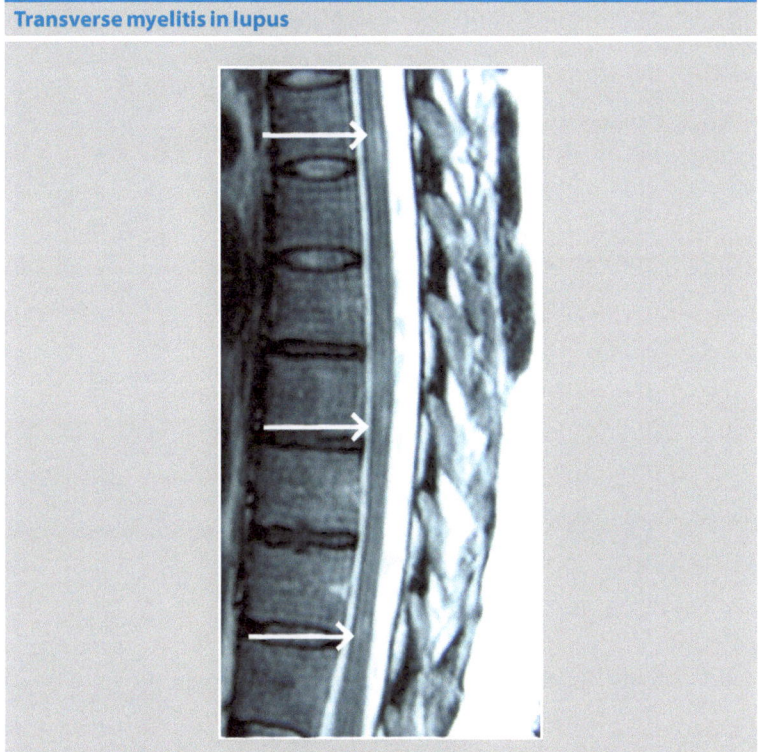

Figure 6.4 Transverse myelitis in lupus. Pale areas in the spinal cord are indicated by arrows. In lupus, this condition is typically caused by inflammation of the spinal cord (shown as pale spots) due to vasculitis and/or the presence of antiphospholipid antibodies.

myasthenia, ocular involvement (including optic neuritis and ischemic lesions). Patients with Hughes syndrome or aPL antibodies are at a greater risk of transient ischemic attacks and stroke.

Treatment

Over the years, aggressive immunosuppressive therapy (eg, pulse cyclophosphamide regimes) and steroids have been used to treat the effects of lupus on the brain, mirroring the practice in lupus nephritis.

More and more, recognition of the role of blood clotting (or 'sludging') in the pathogenesis of lupus with neurological features has lead to the increased use of aspirin, heparin, and warfarin in the management of complex cases.

Chapter 7

Heart and blood vessels

All three layers of the heart can be affected by lupus. Blood vessel involvement is a central feature of the pathology of lupus, causing not just inflammatory small vessel vasculitis, but also thrombosis in the veins and arteries, and later in the course of the disease, accelerated atheroma in a significant number of patients.

Heart

The most common cardiac manifestation is pericarditis (Figure 7.1), usually presenting with sharp central chest pain during a flare of the disease. Inflammation of the pericardium may be accompanied by

Chest CT showing pericardial and pleural effusion

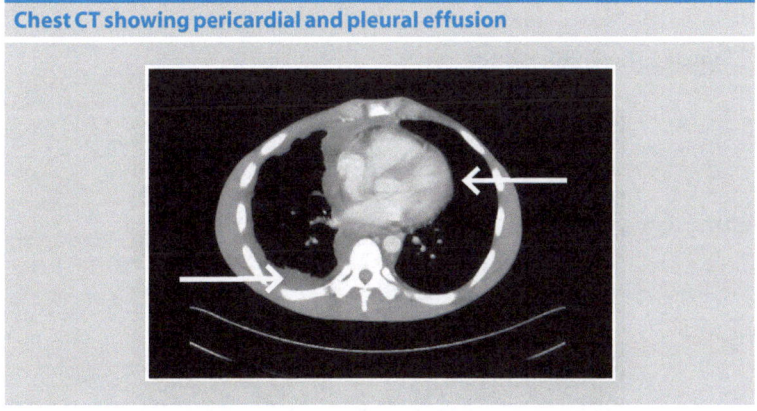

Figure 7.1 Chest CT showing pericardial and pleural effusion. Often related to inflammation. It is estimated that 20–50% of patients with lupus develop pleuritis and/or pericarditis.

pleurisy and, less commonly, by peritonism. The pericarditis occasionally leads to pericardial effusions, although cases of constrictive pericarditis are unusual.

The inflammation of the pericardium generally responds to steroid treatment, with fairly high doses (30–40 mg of prednisolone daily) required to ease the pain. It is said that flares of lupus often follow a similar pattern in an individual and recurrent pericarditis is a feature in some patients. By contrast, inflammatory cardiomyopathy is an unusual feature of lupus. Even in MCTD, where myositis can be prominent, inflammation of the cardiac muscle is unusual.

Historically, one of the earliest known cardiac manifestations of lupus is the thrombotic/vegetative valve lesion known as Libman-Sacks endocarditis (Figure 7.2). This lesion, now recognized as being more of a feature of in Hughes syndrome than of lupus, initially leads to cardiac murmurs and mild echocardiographic changes, but in extreme cases can lead to valve failure. This increases the risk of cerebral emboli and may require treatment with intensive anticoagulation and valve replacement.

Interestingly, valve involvement is much more a feature of Hughes syndrome than of any other prothrombotic disorder and thus echocardiography is an essential part of the investigation of any patient with antiphospholipid antibodies.

Libman-Sacks endocarditis

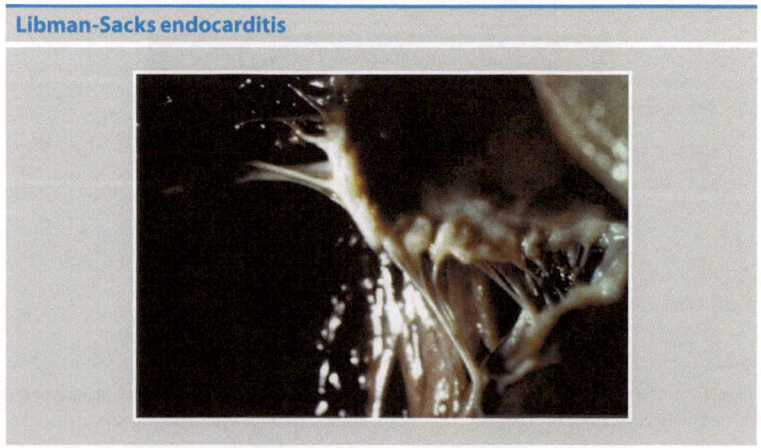

Figure 7.2 Libman-Sacks endocarditis. Libman-Sacks endocarditis is a cardiac manifestation of lupus that causes mulberry-shaped clusters on the ventricular surface of the heart valves.

Atheroma

Coronary artery disease and cardiac ischemia are also recognized as complications of lupus. There are two main causes: aPL antibodies and late atheroma. Patients with aPL antibodies — both those with primary Hughes syndrome and patients with lupus that test positive for aPL antibodies — have been known to have an increased risk of coronary artery thrombosis. For example, testing aPL-positive may increase the risk of heart attack in young women by up to 22 times. Occasionally, myocardial infarction can be acute and fatal.

More subtle arterial thrombotic lesions in Hughes syndrome and patients with lupus that are aPL-positive can lead to cardiac arrhythmias and cardiomyopathy (Figure 7.3). These cases highlight the need in lupus to check aPL status and consider anticoagulant therapy alongside the more routine lupus drugs.

In the long-term patient with lupus, clinicians must be alert to the possible complications of accelerated arterial disease.

Cardiac myoview scan showing cardiac ischemia

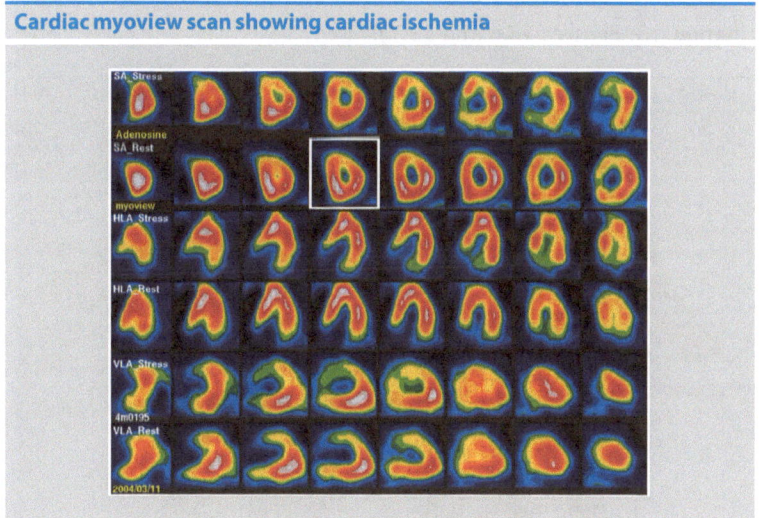

Figure 7.3 **Cardiac myoview scan showing cardiac ischemia.** Results of a cardiac myoview stress test showing cardiac ischemia (as shown in white box). Accelerated atherosclerosis is a feature of lupus and affected patients are at a higher risk of developing ischemic heart disease.

Vasculitis

Vasculitis is a feature of active lupus. The inflammation mainly affects small blood vessels and classical clinical features include small ischemic lesions on the tips of the hands and feet (Figure 7.4 and Figure 7.5). An important diagnostic clue to vasculitis is the presence of small-to-medium sized (1–2 mm) lesions on the elbows.

Other sites where vasculitis may be seen are the nail beds, in the eye on ophthalmoscopic examination (Figure 7.6), and in larger skin ulcers. The other vascular pathology ranges from livedo reticularis (seen especially on the upper arms, wrists, and knees), ischemic lesions that can lead to skin ulcers (Figure 7.7), and in extreme cases, digital limb gangrene.

Thrombosis of larger vessels can include renal artery thrombosis, stroke, myocardial infarction, and occasionally even affect the largest vessels such as the aorta. In lupus, these major arterial lesions are mainly seen in patients that are aPL-positive. A peculiar lesion seen in aPL-positive patients with lupus and in Hughes syndrome is localized stenosis, including renal artery stenosis and celiac artery stenosis (see Chapter 13; Figures 13.6 and 13.7).

Digital vasculitis

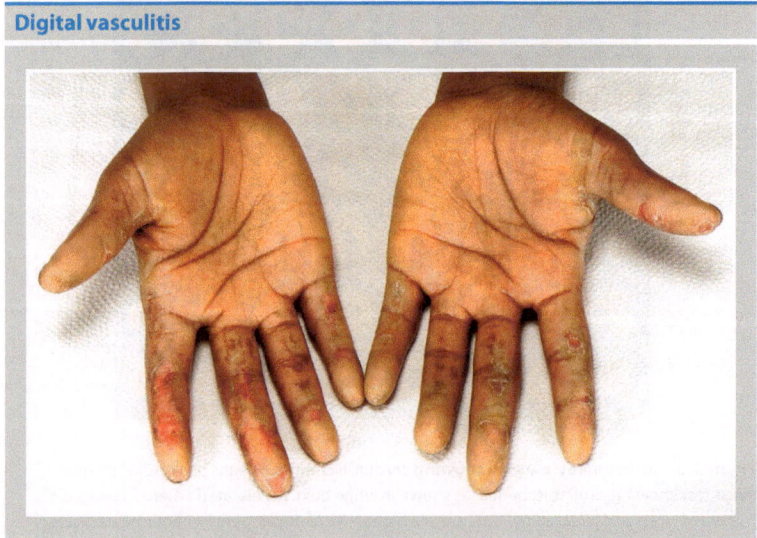

Figure 7.4 Digital vasculitis. Vasculitis of the hands in a patient with lupus, with visible lesions and discoloration.

Vasculitis-associated foot lesions

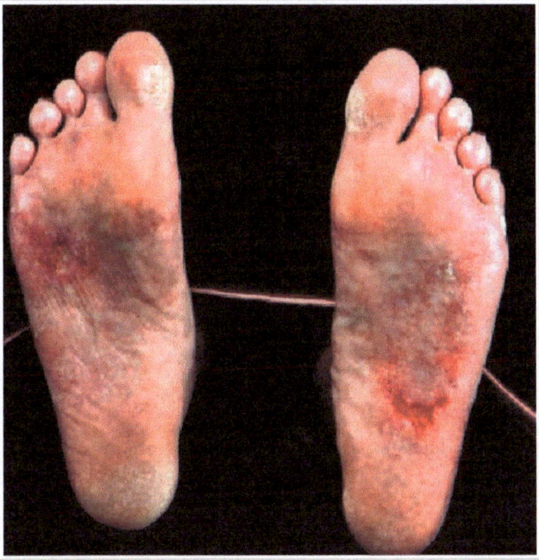

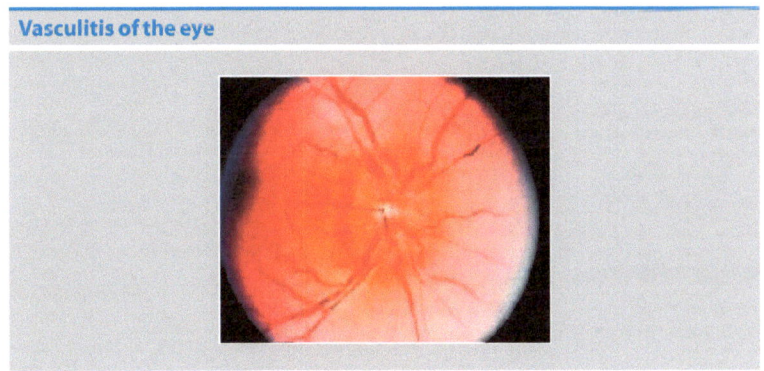

Figure 7.5 Vasculitis-associated foot lesions. Lesions on the foot in a patient with vasculitis. In some patients, lesions may develop into ulcers if left untreated.

Vasculitis of the eye

Figure 7.6 Vasculitis of the eye. Vasculitis of the eye causes inflammation in the small blood vessels of the retina. This may lead to sporadic visual blurring and loss of vision.

Skin ulcers caused by ischemic lesions

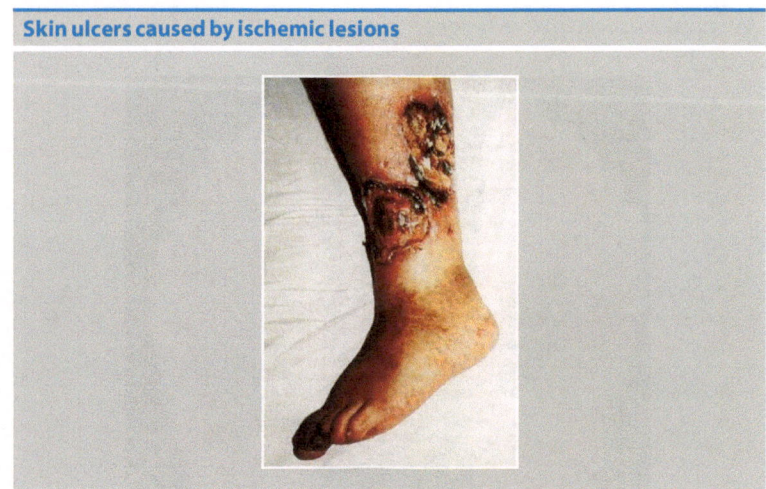

Figure 7.7 Skin ulcers in lupus. Ulcers can result from inflammatory vasculitis and thromboses.

Chapter 8

Liver and gastrointestinal tract

Liver

One of the odd facts about lupus it that the liver is rarely a primary target organ, although the term 'lupoid hepatitis' is used for some forms of autoimmune hepatitis. Thus abnormal liver function tests in a patient with lupus should raise three main alternative diagnoses:

1. Hughes syndrome (with hepatic thrombosis)
2. Drug side-effects (eg, azathiaprine)
3. A secondary diagnosis (eg, infection)

Gastrointestinal tract

Involvement of the gastrointestinal (GI) tract in lupus seems to vary in frequency from continent to continent. For example, this complication is common in South East Asia, but unusual in Western Europe. The three main pathological processes leading to GI involvement are: inflammation (eg, peritonitis), thrombosis (eg, bowel infarction, celiac artery stenosis), or iatrogenic in nature (eg, high-dose steroids, non-steroidal anti-inflammatory drugs).

Abdominal pain is often seen during a lupus flare. Most commonly due to lupus peritonitis, the pain is rarely chronic and usually settles with steroid therapy. Other causes of abdominal pain are bowel ischemia, chronic pancreatitis, and vasculitis. However, an iatrogenic cause, notably due to nonsteroidal anti-inflammatories, is not uncommon.

For patients with Raynaud's phenomenon, esophageal problems, spasms, dysphagia, and reflux esophagitis can be prominent. Sjögren's syndrome, with severe mouth dryness, can also result in dysphagia. As lupus predominately affects a relatively younger age group, gallbladder disease is unusual.

Chapter 9

Blood

Routine blood analysis in lupus can turn up a number of abnormalities including leukopenia (low white blood cell count) (Figure 9.1), anemia, thrombocytopenia, raised erythrocyte sedimentation rate (usually with a normal C-reactive protein level), raised gamma globulin levels, abnormal renal function tests and low vitamin D levels, not to mention the plethora of raised levels of antibodies seen in this disease.

Thrombocytopenia and leukopenia in lupus

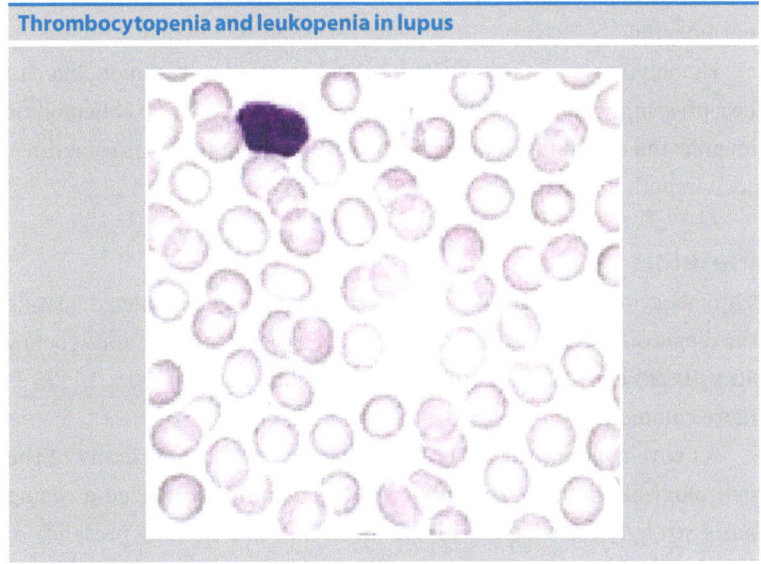

Figure 9.1 Thrombocytopenia and leukopenia in lupus. Blood film showing a lymphocyte but no platelets or other white blood cells.

White blood cells

Leukopenia is common and white blood cell (WBC) counts of 2.0–3.0 x 10^9/L are seen regularly and counts as low as 1.5 or 1.0 x 10^9/L are often seen in otherwise seemingly healthy patients with lupus. The most common cause is neutropenia (though lymphopenia is also frequently seen, especially in patients treated with steroids). Interestingly, despite low WBCs, major infections in these patients are uncommon, presumably because the WBCs which are present function normally.

The clinical difficulty arises in neutropenic patients with lupus on immunosuppressive therapy. Bone marrow examination may be needed to make a correct diagnosis. However, it is an interesting fact that in many neutropenic patients with lupus, WBCs increase when treatment is stepped up (even with immunosuppressive therapy).

Red cells

Anemia in lupus is most commonly either iron-deficient (often due to nonsteroidal medication) or due to chronic inflammation (normochromic normocytic).

Hemolytic anemia (often Coombs'-positive) is less common, but can be a presenting manifestation of the disease. A combination of hemolytic anemia and thrombocytopenic purpura (Evans syndrome) is sometimes seen in both lupus and Hughes syndrome.

Platelets

Thrombocytopenia is a well known feature of lupus, sometimes antedating the diagnosis of lupus by years. Although very low platelet counts (below 10 x 10^9/L) can be seen, mild thrombocytopenia (90–100 x 10^9/L) is more common.

As with some of the other features of lupus (such as many of the neurological features), thrombocytopenia is now recognized as being more strongly associated with Hughes syndrome and the presence of circulating aPL antibodies.

PART THREE

Diagnosis and treatment

Chapter 10

Diagnosing lupus

Lupus is a condition where a single test is almost diagnostic; high titres of double stranded anti-DNA antibodies (dsDNA) are rarely, if ever, seen in any other condition. The only other condition which sometimes gives diagnostic difficulty is Sjögren's syndrome (see Chapter 12), where high titers of anti-nuclear antibodies can lead (usually for technical reasons) to 'borderline' positive anti dsDNA titers.

Statistically, lupus primarily affects young woman (9:1 female: male ratio), thus it is vanishingly rare to see a new case of lupus in a fifty year old male, for example (Figure 10.1).

An unusual case: a male patient with lupus

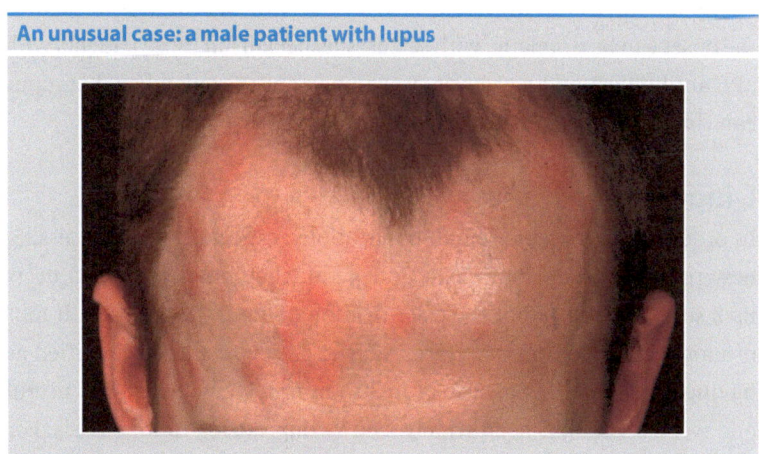

Figure 10.1 An unusual case: a male patient with lupus. Lupus does affect males but accounts for less than 10% of total cases. The disease does not appear to differ in presentation or severity.

Clinical clues

Skin

The 'classical' butterfly rash on the cheeks and bridge of the nose is, in fact, seen in less than half of all patients. Skin rashes, while common, can present in many forms and on different parts of the body. Examination should always include inspecting the elbows for small red spots or blisters, as the elbows are a favored site of vasculitis but uncommon in other diseases with rashes. Other important rash sites are the eyebrows, the V-neck, the scalp (alopecia is a major diagnostic clue), palms, and soles of feet.

Malaise

Lupus often presents gradually and can result in delayed diagnosis. Fatigue is the most common symptom, with flu-like aches and pains (but no swelling) being prominent. Chest discomfort (usually from pleurisy) is common, as is weight loss, fever, and lymphadenopathy.

Neuropsychiatric features

Neuropsychiatric features including headache, depression, and phobias can be prominent, especially in the early stages of the disease. Occasionally, the onset can be dramatic, with seizures (especially in those patients with aPL antibodies) and psychosis. It is important to remember that lupus can flare or present for the first time in the early puerperium.

Diagnostic criteria

In order to regularise research publications, especially those assessing new treatments, the American College of Rheumatology (ACR) drew up a set of 11 criteria for the classification of lupus (Table 10.1). If four or more of these criteria are present, the patient could be classified as having lupus for the purpose of inclusion in a study. Sadly this useful and worthy goal has been widely, and wrongly, used for diagnosis. For example, a person with only three criteria may be excluded from lupus diagnosis. The ACR criteria have also been taken up by patient groups and appears in general literature.

1997 update of the 1982 American College of Rheumatology revised criteria for classification of systemic lupus erythematosus

Criterion	Definition
1. Malar rash	Fixed erythema, (flat or raised), over the malar eminences, tending to spare the nasolabial folds
2. Discoid rash	Erythematous raised patches with adherent keratotic scaling and follicular plugging; atrophic scarring may occur in older lesions
3. Photosensitivity	Skin rash as a result of unusual reaction to sunlight, by patient history or physician observation
4. Oral ulcers	Oral or nasopharyngeal ulceration, usually painless, observed by physician
5. Nonerosive arthritis	Involving 2 or more peripheral joints, characterized by tenderness, swelling, or effusion
6. Pleuritis or Pericarditis	a. Pleuritis: convincing history of pleuritic pain or rubbing heard by a physician or evidence of pleural effusion **OR** b. Pericarditis: documented by electrocardigram or rub or evidence of pericardial effusion
7. Renal disorder	a. Persistent proteinuria > 0.5 grams per day or > than 3+ if quantitation not performed **OR** b. Cellular casts: may be red cell, hemoglobin, granular, tubular, or mixed
8. Neurologic disorder	a. Seizures: in the absence of offending drugs or known metabolic derangements; (eg, uremia, ketoacidosis, or electrolyte imbalance) **OR** b. Psychosis: in the absence of offending drugs or known metabolic derangements, (eg, uremia, ketoacidosis, or electrolyte imbalance)
9. Hematologic disorder	a. Hemolytic anemia-with reticulocytosis **OR** b. Leukopenia: < 4,000/mm³ on ≥ 2 occasions **OR** c. Lyphopenia: < 1,500/ mm³ on ≥ 2 occasions **OR** d. Thrombocytopenia: <100,000/ mm³ in the absence of offending drugs
10. Immunology	a. Anti-DNA: antibody to native DNA in abnormal titer **OR** b. Anti-Sm: presence of antibody to Sm nuclear antigen **OR** c. Positive finding of antiphospholipid antibodies on: 1. an abnormal serum level of IgG or IgM anticardiolipin antibodies 2. a positive test result for lupus anticoagulant using a standard method 3. a false-positive test result for at least 6 months confirmed by Treponema pallidum immobilization or fluorescent treponemal antibody absorption test
11. Positive antinuclear antibody	An abnormal titer of antinuclear antibody by immunofluorescence or an equivalent assay at any point in time and in the absence of drugs

Table 10.1 1997 update of the 1982 American College of Rheumatology revised criteria for classification of systemic lupus erythematosus. Disease criteria used for lupus classification. If a patient has 4 or more of 11 criteria, it is considered likely that the patient has lupus.

Clearly, for the physician considering a possible diagnosis of lupus, these criteria are extremely restrictive, as one could correctly diagnose lupus in a patient with a butterfly rash, seizures, hair loss, and nephritis, but would potentially misdiagnose dozens of patients that display less 'classical' symptoms.

Some years ago, our group drew up a list of criteria which might prove useful as pointers towards a diagnosis of lupus (Table 10.2). While many of the features on this 'alternative criteria' list are not specific, collectively two or three positive in a young woman with ongoing malaise could be suggestive of possible lupus.

Laboratory tests

There are several key tests in a patient with suspected lupus: anti-dsDNA, full blood count, erythrocyte sedimentation rate (ESR), C-reactive protein (CRP), electrolytes, and urinalysis in particular.

Anti-DNA and other antibodies

The hallmark of lupus is the frequency and breadth of non-organ specific antibodies such as anti-DNA, anti-Smith (Sm), anti-Ro, and anti-RNP. Organ-specific antibodies such as thyroid and celiac antibodies (more common in Sjögren's syndrome) are rather unusual.

The 'screening' test for lupus is the anti-nuclear antibody (ANA) test. This test potentially picks up a variety of non organ–specific antibodies (Figure 10.2A and B). Over 90% of patients with lupus are ANA-positive, usually in titers higher than 1 in 80. Other diseases, notably Sjögren's syndrome, rheumatoid arthritis, and other autoimmune conditions, can show ANA positivity. Rarely, drug reactions can show lupus-like features and cause a patient to test ANA-positive (drug-induced lupus).

Since their discovery some 40 years ago, anti-DNA antibody tests have turned out to be one of the most specific in the whole of medicine. It is extremely rare for false positives to occur for any other disease.

St Thomas' alternative criteria for lupus diagnosis

1.	Teenage "growing pains"	"Growing pains" in the UK is a label widely used for joint pains in teenagers and seems to cover a spectrum of rheumatology from arthritis through to lupus
2.	Teenage migraine	Headache, cluster headache, and migraine can be encountered and a strong history of teenage migraine may be of lupus significance, either at the time or subsequently
3.	Teenage 'glandular fever'	Prolonged teenage 'glandular fever' is a diagnosis often wrongly applied and prolonged periods off school in many patients with lupus is a recurrent issue
4.	Severe reaction to insect bites	A common feature in many patients with lupus. Not only are they susceptible to insect bites but often reactions are severe and prolonged, as the skin is a major organ affected by lupus
5.	Recurrent miscarriages	Lupus itself does not seem to be a cause of recurrent miscarriage but when the antiphospholipid syndrome is present, recurrent spontaneous fetal loss can occur
6.	Premenstrual tension	Although difficult to quantify, it is believed that significant premenstrual syndrome flare is sufficiently prominent in lupus to be included in this list. All rheumatic diseases are clinically influenced by the menstrual cycle
7.	Septrin allergy	Adverse reactions to septrin are quite common in lupus and the clinical onset of the disease may coincide with their use
8.	Agoraphobia	Agoraphobia/claustrophobia are often present at a time when lupus disease is active. A history of these conditions (including panic attacks), can be protracted, lasting for months or even years. In many cases, the history is not volunteered or the episodes are in the interim and considered unrelated to lupus
9.	Finger flexor tendonitis	Arthralgia and tenosynovitis are common features in lupus and although not specific, the finding of mild to moderate ten-finger flexor synovitis is a useful pointer in the presence of other lupus features. It is subtly yet significantly different in pattern to other arthritic diseases
10.	Family history of autoimmune disease	As the genetics and statistics of the various autoimmune diseases become better defined, the strength of a particular family history will become more precise. The family history is important, as lupus can be genetically determined
11.	Dry Schirmer's test	A "bone dry" Schirmer's test (testing levels of eye moisture) points towards Sjögren's syndrome and in the patient with vague or nonspecific symptoms, it is a very useful test
12.	Borderline C4	Genetic complement deficiencies have been known to be associated with lupus for over three decades and in the diagnostically difficult patient, especially where a family history is present, borderline C4 levels can be significant indicators
13.	Normal CRP with raised ESR	A very low CRP in an otherwise inflammatory situation is strongly supportive of lupus or primary Sjögren's syndrome
14.	Lymphopenia	In the patient with nonspecific complaints and unremarkable blood tests, a borderline or low lymph count can be overlooked. It can be common in lupus and is certainly worth inclusion among minor criteria to assist in making a diagnosis

Table 10.2 St Thomas' alternative criteria for lupus diagnosis. Ten clinical and four investigative criteria based on clinical experience. CRP, C-reactive protein; ESR, erythrocyte sedimentation rate.

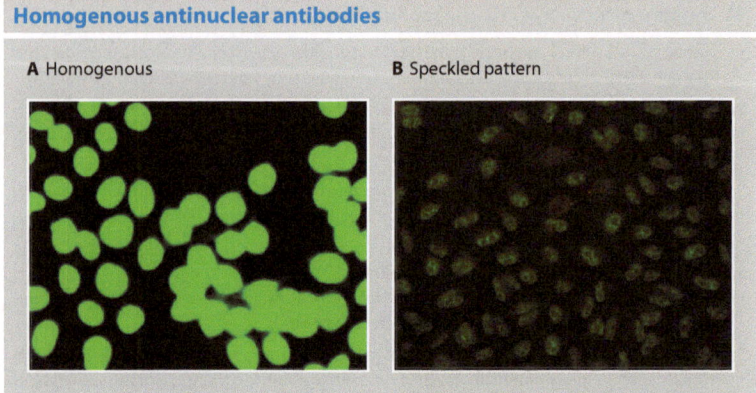

Homogenous antinuclear antibodies

A Homogenous   **B** Speckled pattern

Figure 10.2 A and B Homogenous antinuclear antibodies. Antinuclear antibodies (ANA) are observed in over 90% of patients with lupus. The test screens for auto-antibodies in the bloodstream, and the pattern and titer of the results are then used to determine the origin. They are also seen in other related conditions such as Sjögren's and scleroderma.

Other antibodies

Extractable nuclear antibodies is the name given to a collection of anti-nuclear and anti-cytoplasmic antibodies identified in lupus. Some of the more important in lupus are:

- **Anti-Sm:** Fairly specific for lupus, but less diagnostically useful than anti-DNA. (Named after a patient called Smith).
- **Anti-RNP:** Seen in mixed connective tissue disease (see Chapter 14) and lupus. Strongly associated with Raynaud's phenomenon.
- **Anti-Ro and Anti-La:** Associated with Sjögren's, with photosensitivity and cutaneous rashes, notably SCLE (see Chapter 3). Also associated with rare fetal problems of neonatal lupus rash and congenital heart block.
- **Anti-C1q:** Not in widespread use, but said to be a useful marker for renal disease in lupus.

Antiphospholipid antibodies

Antiphospholipid (aPL) antibodies are generally measured by two tests: anticardiolipin antibodies and the so-called 'lupus anticoagulant'. Both tests are required, as some sera only demonstrate positivity in one of the two tests (Table 10.3). In recent years, a third serum test (anti-beta 2 glycoprotein 1) has been added, but is not yet in widespread use.

Laboratory results from a patient with aPL-positive Hughes syndrome	
Antibody	**aPL result**
LA	Positive
aCL (IgM/IgG)	Medium to high titer
B₂ GPI (IgM/IgG)	Medium to high titer

Table 10.3 Laboratory results from a patient with aPL-positive Hughes syndrome. Positive lupus anticoagulant (LA) or anticardiolipin (aCL) antibodies and/or B2 glycoprotein I (B₂GPI) in medium to high titers at least twice (twelve weeks apart) are included in criteria for Hughes syndrome. aPL, antiphospholipid.

Testing for aPL antibodies is one of the single most important diagnostic procedures in lupus, as it pinpoints patients with lupus that are more prone to arterial and venous thrombosis.

Full blood count

Leukopenia, anemia, and (occasionally) thrombocytopenia are features of lupus (see Figure 9.1). In the commonly faced differential diagnosis of lupus versus infection, the WBC count can be a helpful diagnostic tool, as WBC count is low in lupus but high in infections.

Complement levels

During flares of lupus, it is common for complement levels (usually C3 and C4 are measured) to fall. However, an interpretation of this can be flawed, as a number of patients with lupus have various genetic complement deficiencies that can lead, for example, to a permanently low C4 level.

C-reactive protein

CRP levels are generally low in lupus but rise when an infection is present. In the management of febrile patients with lupus, the CRP test is an extremely valuable guide to distinguishing between a lupus flare or an infection.

Urinalysis and electrolytes

The routine monitoring of any patient with lupus must include assessment of renal function by measuring urea, creatinine, and electrolytes. In addition, measuring serum albumin will give a guide to the degree of proteinuria, if present. Proteinuria is the most common early marker of lupus renal involvement, with active urine sediment suggesting more active renal disease. Thus, a routine part of any lupus consultation is urinalysis.

Other investigations

X-rays, echocardiography, doppler, dual-emission X-ray absorptiometry (DEXA), MRI, and angiography are all part of the diagnostic armamentarium in lupus.

Chapter 11

Treatment

One of the major advances in the management of lupus has been the move towards more conservative treatment. Gone is long-term use of high-dose steroids for all, with a graded and more individualised approach now recommended instead.

General management

As many patients with lupus are photosensitive, avoidance of excessive ultraviolet (UV) light is advisable (Figure 11.1). The most harmful UV light to a patient with lupus is that given out during the midday hours. Sunscreens are moderately effective but not totally preventative to sensitive lupus skin.

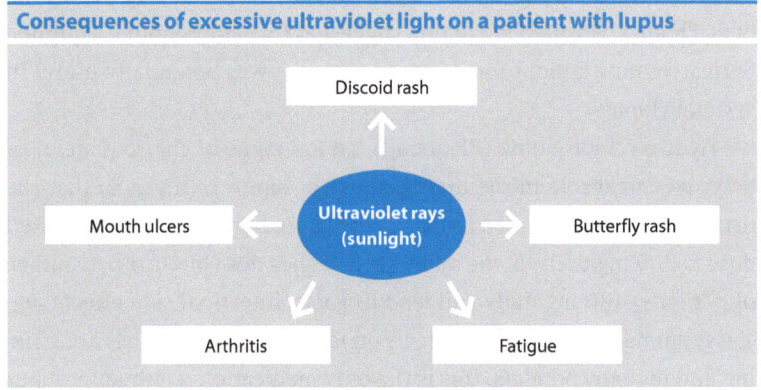

Figure 11.1 Consequences of excessive ultraviolet light on a patient with lupus. Ultraviolet light (especially around midday) can cause a flare in lupus symptoms.

Vitamin D

Is it well understood that Vitamin D, a hormone, is important for bone strength. However, it is now known to have an important role in immune protection (Figure 11.2). Increasingly, Vitamin D supplementation is being advocated in lupus. Vitamin D levels can be measured using a simple blood test and will likely become a standard investigation in lupus.

Diet

There is not currently a specific diet recommended for patients with lupus, although many have been advocated.

Middle-aged patients with lupus have been found to have a higher tendency towards atheroma. The reasons for this are still being investigated and suspects include steroids, inflammation, and aPL antibodies, among others. Thus, in terms of practical therapeutics, lipid/cholesterol checks and dietary measures are important. Statins are increasingly used at an early stage in patients with lupus who have marginally raised cholesterol levels.

Drug therapy

Plaquenil

Quinine, derived from the cinchona tree of South America, has long been known for its therapeutic properties, especially in the management of fever, joint pains and fatigue. Just over a century ago, Dr Payne of St Thomas' Hospital in London suggested that chloroquine, a quinine derivative now famous for its use in malaria, was potentially useful in systemic lupus.

Hydroxychloroquine (Plaquenil), an analogue of chloroquine, now plays a central role in the management of lupus, so much so that the drug has become regarded as maintenance therapy. The commonly used dose is 200 mg daily. Some advocate a higher dose but in a percentage of patients, 400 mg daily can lead to gastrointestinal side effects (eg, 'gassy stomach'). The drug's effects on fatigue and skin rashes are striking and in many patients, this is the only medication required for lupus management. Plaquenil is safe in pregnancy and, at a low dose, is not toxic to the retina. However, patients should be informed that smoking reduces the drug's therapeutic effect.

Metabolism of vitamin D

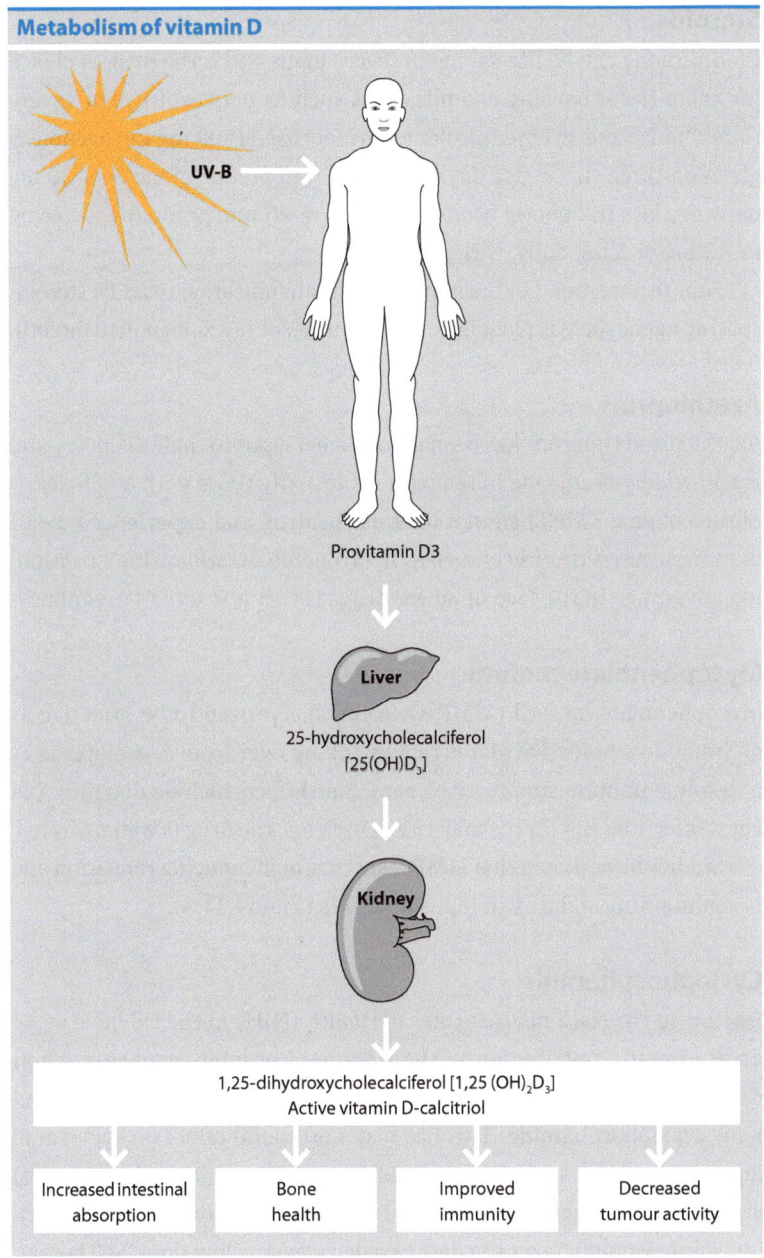

UV-B

Provitamin D3

Liver

25-hydroxycholecalciferol
[25(OH)D$_3$]

Kidney

1,25-dihydroxycholecalciferol [1,25 (OH)$_2$D$_3$]
Active vitamin D-calcitriol

| Increased intestinal absorption | Bone health | Improved immunity | Decreased tumour activity |

Figure 11.2 Metabolism of vitamin D. A pictorial representation of the metabolism of vitamin D (cholecalciferol). Low vitamin D levels may cause T lymphocyte dysfunction, which can lead to immune disorders.

Steroids

Prednisolone can be life-saving in severe lupus and is the drug of choice for acute flares causing complications such as pericarditis. For severe flares, 'pulse' methyl prednisolone is widely used (500 mg intravenously given on three successive days). Doses of oral prednisolone over 30 mg daily are less frequently used and a dose of 20 mg, gradually lowering to 7.5 mg or 5 mg daily, is the aim.

Failure to respond to the lower doses is an indication to add a steroid-sparing agent such as plaquenil, azathioprine, or mycophenolate mofetil.

Azathioprine

Azathioprine (Imuran) has been used to treat lupus for half a century and is still widely used. One in ten patients (usually those with a deficiency of the enzyme TMPT) cannot tolerate the drug and experience nausea or more severe side effects such as neutropenia. Azathioprine's continuing advantage in the face of newer drugs is that it is safe in pregnancy.

Mycophenolate mofetil

Mycophenolate mofetil (MMF, Cellcept) has proved to be effective as an immunosuppressive and is rapidly taking over from azathioprine as a first-line immunosuppressive agent. Side effects include diarrhea and chest infections but for the majority of patients, the drug is well tolerated.

Studies have shown that MMF is successful in inducing remission and in maintaining stability in lupus nephritis (Figure 11.3).

Cyclophosphamide

Doctors at the National Institutes of Health (NIH) in the US have made an enormous contribution to the treatment of lupus nephritis. Their careful studies introduced the 'NIH regime' of regular pulses of intravenous cyclophosphamide. This has had a profound effect on survival in lupus nephritis but had a high incidence of infections (including shingles) and a high incidence of ovarian failure, a disaster in a disease affecting young women. Over the past two decades, the low dose 'St Thomas' Hospital regime' showed lower doses (eg, 500 mg cyclophosphamide every two weeks for six pulses) was equally effective but with far fewer

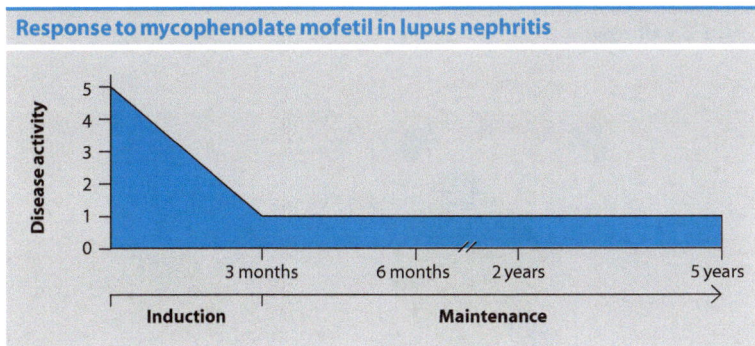

Figure 11.3 Response to mycophenolate mofetil in lupus nephritis. Mycophenate mofetil is an immunosuppressive agent used to induce remission and provide long term (>5 years) maintenance in active lupus nephritis.

side effects. This low dose regime is now being taken up all over Europe and is known as the 'Euro-Lupus' regime (Figure 11.4).

Anti B cell agents

This is the era of the monoclonal antibodies, which are immunosuppressive agents that allow a more focused attack on the mediators of the disease, such as the B cell (Figure 11.5).

For example, rituximab, an anti-B cell agent, is already in wide usage for severe lupus. Initial experience is very positive both in efficiency and tolerance. Belimumab (Benlysta®), an agent focused on a B cell marker looks equally promising and has recently overcome most of the hurdles

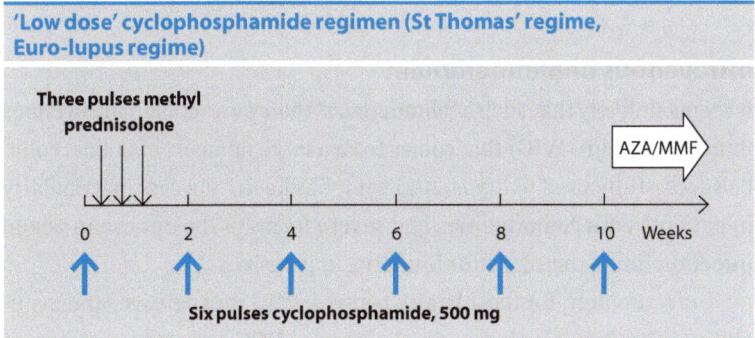

Figure 11.4 'Low dose' cyclophosphamide regimen (St Thomas' regime), (Euro-lupus regime). Low dose cyclophosphamide has few side effects and does not appear to cause infections or infertility. It is as effective as higher doses (eg, NIH regime).

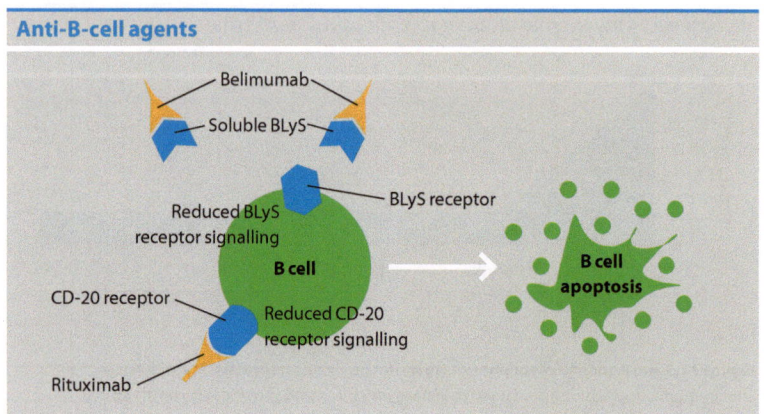

Figure 11.5 Anti-B-cell agents. A reduction in BLyS or CD-20 signalling in B cells promotes apoptosis and reduces inflammation. Belimumab blocks binding of soluble BLyS to its receptors. BLyS, B lymphocyte stimulator.

to become a recognized drug prescribed specifically for the treatment of lupus. So far, this is the only drug which has been approved by the Food and Drug Administration in the US and European Medicines Agency in Europe for the treatment of lupus. Preliminary results are very promising as a specific therapy targeting antibody proliferation, and in clinical trials, levels of anticardiolipin antibodies were also reduced. This drug has opened a new chapter for patients who were previously bombarded with corticosteroids and nonspecific immunosuppressive drugs. At long last a number of new agents (abatacept, atacicept, and epratuzumab to name a few) are on the horizon for lupus treatment.

Intravenous immunoglobulin

It seems unlikely that such a 'blunderbuss' therapy as pooled intravenous immunoglobulin (IVIG) that comes from a large numbers of donors could be successfully used in lupus. And yet it has been a success, particularly in patients with comorbidities and severe forms of the disease in whom infection limits the scope for immunosuppressives.

Unfortunately, for most health centres, IVIG is expensive, and availability is limited. Furthermore, the normal IVIG treatment consists of five days of intravenous infusions that must take place within a hospital, which is a major consideration. Perhaps an alternative treatment will come from the splitting off of the active components for use against specific antibody-mediated diseases.

Plasma exchange

In 1973, we published a study in *The Lancet* describing the first study of plasmapheresis in lupus. It was not a particularly good study and unfortunately, there have been few good studies since. In theory, plasmapheresis (the spinning down of blood allowing the removal of 'bad' antibodies) has huge potential. It is still used, but mainly in intensive care units, and appears in anecdotal data in cases such as catastrophic Hughes syndrome. Results are encouraging but further investigation is needed.

PART FOUR

Lupus-like disorders

Chapter 12

Sjögren's syndrome

In 1905, Henrik Sjögren, a Swedish ophthalmologist, described a triad of clinical features consisting of dry eyes, dry mouth and aches and pains. In the past 40 years or so, the syndrome has come to be recognized as not only as a common and important condition, but a syndrome occupying a central pivotal place amongst autoimmune diseases (Figure 12.1).

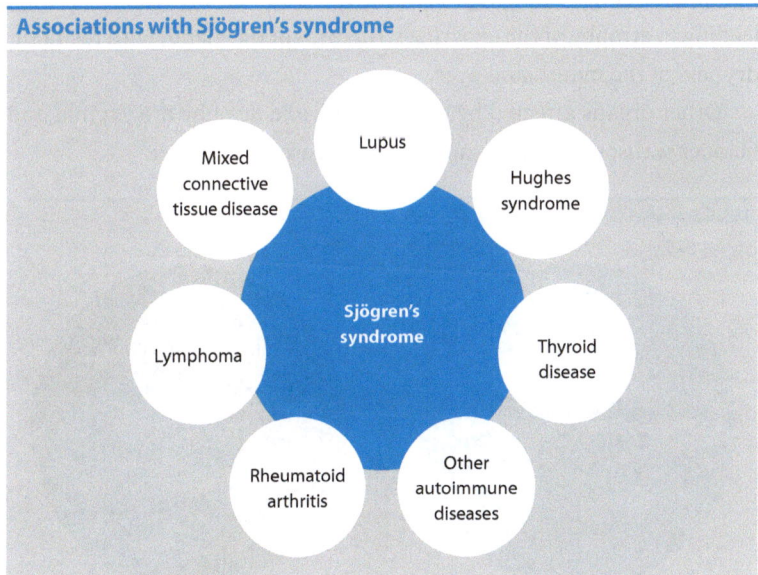

Associations with Sjögren's syndrome

Figure 12.1 Associations with Sjögren's syndrome. Diseases and conditions associated with Sjögren's syndrome. The syndrome tends to be associated with other autoimmune and connective tissue diseases.

In many ways, Sjögren's is considered the 'older first cousin' of lupus, as there is a similar proliferation of auto-antibodies (in particular ANA), the clinical features of fatigue, aches, pains, and occasional sun sensitivity.

The main differences between the diseases are that Sjögren's affects an older age group, generally has fewer life-threatening features, and patients with Sjögren's have a tendency to produce both organ specific antibodies (eg, thyroid) as well as non-organ specific antibodies (eg, ANA).

It is now customary to classify Sjögren's syndrome as 'primary' but when accompanied by other clear cut diagnoses such as rheumatoid arthritis, it is classified as 'secondary' (Figure 12.2).

Pathology

The main pathological finding in Sjögren's syndrome is a lymphoid infiltrate in the exocrine glands, notably the salivary and lachrymal glands, but also extending elsewhere. The initial stage is of a focal infiltration, but in later stages the lymphoid infiltrate can become overwhelming, leading to atrophy of the exocrine structures of the gland, with resultant dryness of the mouth and eyes.

Other organs affected by the infiltrate and atrophy are vaginal and bladder walls, esophagus, and the upper respiratory tract.

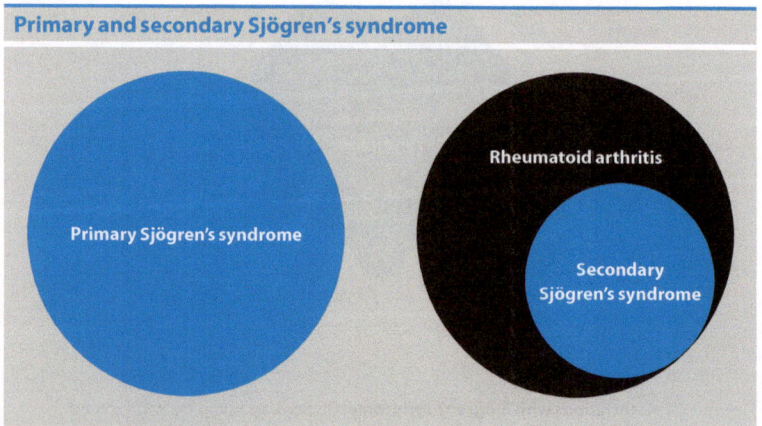

Primary and secondary Sjögren's syndrome

Primary Sjögren's syndrome

Rheumatoid arthritis

Secondary Sjögren's syndrome

Figure 12.2 Primary and secondary Sjögren's syndrome. Sjögren's syndrome is considered primary when it occurs alone; when associated with another disease (eg, rheumatoid arthritis), it is termed secondary.

Clinical features

General

The most common age of onset is generally later than that of lupus, usually in the 4th or 5th decade. As well as dry eyes and mouth, there may be considerable fatigue. Myalgia and arthritis are frequent, though commonly occur without joint swelling. There may be morning stiffness and, in some patients, a history of photosensitivity. Lymphadenopathy, particularly in the neck, is intermittent. In some patients, splenomegaly (a tippable spleen) is noted.

It is important to remember the clinical features of the conditions associated with Sjögren's, including Hughes syndrome (headache, migraine, balance disturbance, and transient ischemic attack) and hypothyroidism (constipation, cold sensitivity, skin changes, weight gain and sluggish reflexes) (Figure 12.3).

Allergies (including food allergy) are also a strong feature of the condition. For example, in the years when gold salts were used in the treatment of rheumatoid arthritis, allergic reactions were twice as common in rheumatoid athritis patients with associated Sjögren's as in those without.

One common feature is an allergy to Septrin, a sulphur-containing antibiotic now rarely used. Septrin allergy was such a regular feature in the past history of Sjögren's patients that it became something of a diagnostic criterion.

Eye

Although dryness of the eyes is one of the pivotal features of the syndrome, many patients do not notice or complain of it. A more common complaint is of irritation or scratchiness, which is often put down to allergy or hay fever. In others, there may be a history of 'stickiness' of the eyes in the morning, photophobia, or difficulty with contact lenses. Later stages can include corneal ulceration.

Mouth and gastrointestinal tract

A dry mouth is possibly the most common complaint in Sjögren's, with many patients having to take a jug of water to bed with them. Both the quantity as well as the quality of the saliva produced by the infiltrated

Features of Sjögren's syndrome

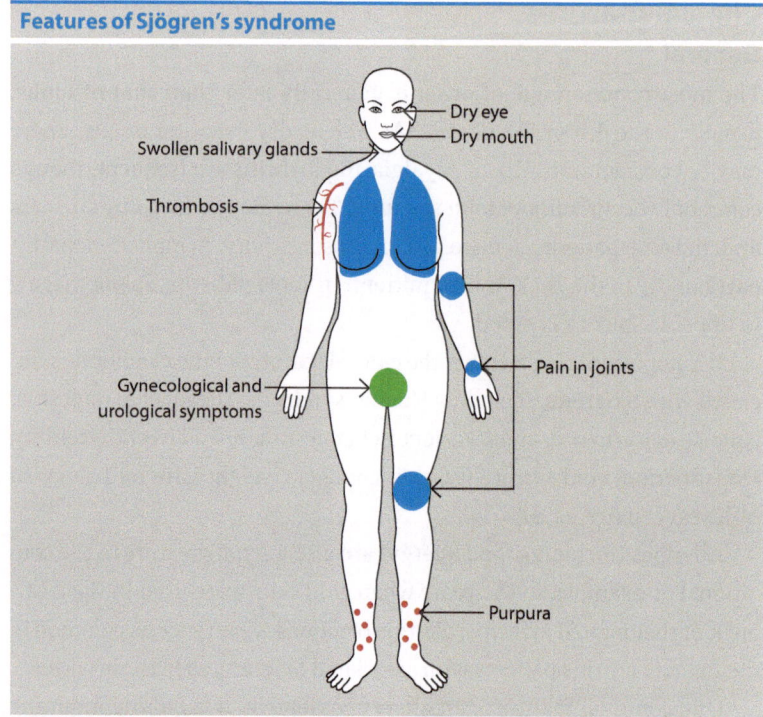

Figure 12.3 Features of Sjögren's syndrome. Symptoms of Sjögren's disease include dry eyes, dry mouth, swollen salivary glands, vasculitis, pulmonary symptoms, joint pain, and gynecological/urological problems. Sjögren's syndrome is a chronic autoimmune disorder in which tear and saliva production is impaired.

salivary glands is poor. In the early stages of Sjögren's, the parotid and submandibular glands can become swollen, either intermittently, or chronically, and in some cases significant parotid gland swelling can lead to a characteristic 'hamster' or 'marmoset' facies.

Poor saliva leads to poor dental hygiene, and gum and dental problems are common in Sjögren's and require vigilant dental care.

If the mouth dryness extends into the esophagus, swallowing dry foods is made even more difficult. It is possible that poor mucus protection in the stomach mucosa might render Sjögren's patients more at risk from anti-inflammatory drug-induced gastritis.

Vagina and bladder

Vaginitis sicca is a problem in many patients, leading to dyspareunia, thrush, and other vaginal problems. Somewhat underestimated has been the problem of recurrent cystitis in Sjögren's – in some cases urethral symptoms; in others, more serious interstitial cystitis.

Kidney

Renal tubular acidosis, and occasionally other renal tubular defects, have long been recognized as a complication of Sjögren's, notably those patients with very high globulin levels. Occasionally, the renal involvement is that of interstitial nephritis (Figure 12.4). Glomerular nephritis has been reported but is rare.

Nervous system

Trigeminal neuralgia, a neuropathic disorder that causes short, stabbing bursts of facial pain, is commonly seen in Sjögren's. It is also a feature of Hughes syndrome but the exact inter-relationships of these two syndromes and trigeminal neuralgia are not yet certain. Other cranial neuropathies, as well as peripheral neuropathy, are sometimes seen. Central nervous system involvement is reported, but the complications described (stroke and atypical multiple sclerosis, for example), may be more strongly associated with Hughes syndrome rather than to Sjögren's *per se*.

The same may be true for the balance problems sometimes seen in Sjögren's, some of which may be secondary to the associated conditions of hypothyroidism or Hughes syndrome.

Blood

As with lupus, borderline neutropenia is a common feature of Sjögren's. In some cases, persistent moderately severe neutropenia (eg, 1.0–2.0 x 10^9 WBC/L) is seen with little in the way of infections (see Figure 9.1). Thrombocytopenia and hemolytic anemia are well reported but unusual.

Interstitial nephritis in Sjögren's disease

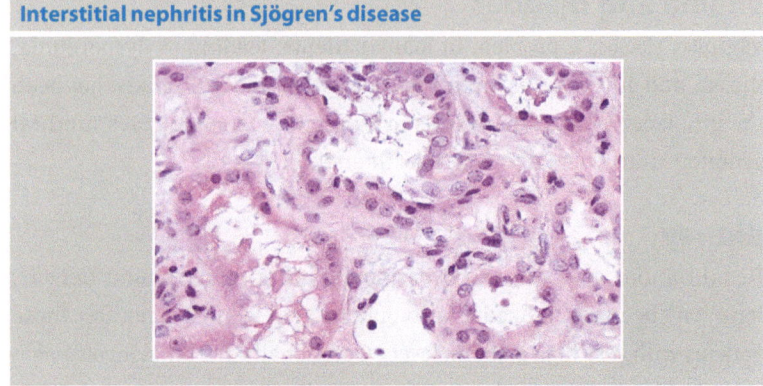

Figure 12.4 Interstitial nephritis in Sjögren's disease. A renal biopsy specimen showing tubular damage in a kidney of a patient with Sjögren's syndrome. Interstitial nephritis is a kidney disorder involving inflammation of kidney tubules, which can affect the kidney function and inhibit waste filtration.

Many Sjögren's patients run a persistently raised ESR (eg, over 40mm/hour); indeed Sjögren's is one of the more prominent causes of prolonged unexplained raised ESR. Interestingly, as in the case of lupus, the CRP may remain low even in the face of a raised ESR.

Purpura

A small number of Sjögren's patients notice intermittent purpuric lesions on the lower legs. These often appear after unusual exercise or long-haul flights. In some patients, the frequency and severity of the purpura can lead to chronic discolouration of the legs (usually below the knees). In extreme cases, peripheral neuropathy can result from the purpura-induced ischemia.

Other autoimmune diseases

Other autoimmune diseases, notably Hashimoto's thyroiditis, idiopathic hypothyroidism and Addison's disease, are known to be associated with Sjögren's. Others include pernicious anemia, celiac disease, rheumatoid arthritis and multiple sclerosis. Somewhat surprisingly, the strengths of some of these associations are not fully elucidated and some may be underestimated. For example, routine Schirmer tear testing for Sjögren's is probably not practised in many cases of multiple sclerosis.

Malignancy

Non-Hodgkin's lymphoma (NHL) is increased in frequency in all autoimmune conditions, but particularly in primary Sjögren's (Figure 12.5); there is a 44-fold increase compared with the general population, especially in cases with persistently enlarged parotids and chronic lymphadenopathy. However, the tendency to NHL may not be a feature of the mild version of Sjögren's that is usually associated with rheumatoid arthritis.

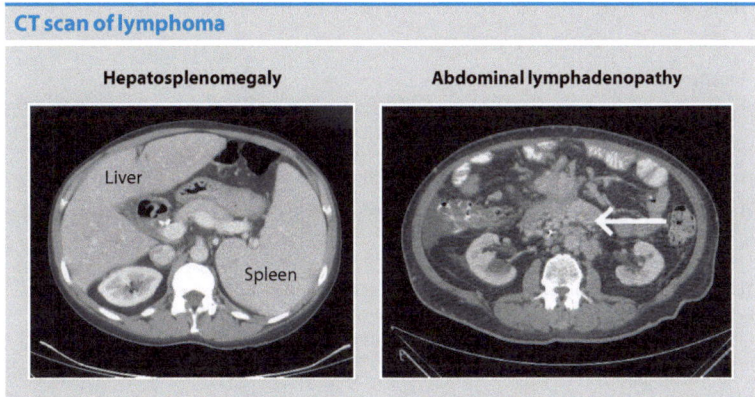

CT scan of lymphoma

Hepatosplenomegaly   Abdominal lymphadenopathy

Figure 12.5 CT scan of lymphoma. A CT scan of patient with lymphoma showing enlarged liver, spleen and abdominal lymph nodes (arrowed). A small number of Ro-positive patients with Sjögren's develop Non Hodgkin's lymphoma.

Diagnosis

Table 12.1 lists the main diagnostic features of Sjögren's syndrome.

Schirmer's tear test

The Schirmer's tear test, although somewhat simple, is a surprisingly useful clinical aide (Figure 12.6).

A sterile, standardised strip of blotting paper (Schirmer paper) is hooked over the lower eyelid and left for 5 minutes. In normal eyes, the irritation caused by the paper soaks the blotter in seconds. In Sjögren's, it is often totally dry. Conventionally, wetting of under 15mm is considered an abnormal ("dry") Schirmer's test. The major benefit of the test is that it generally gives a clear answer, especially as, somewhat surprisingly, diuretics, antihistamines and older age have little drying effect on a Schirmer's test.

The main diagnostic features of Sjögren's syndrome
Routine tests
Raised ESR/normal CRP
WBC normal or low
Hyperglobulinemia (polyclonal)
Immunology
Positive ANA 60–80%
Positive anti-Ro and anti-La 50–60%
Negative anti dsDNA
Positive rheumatoid factor 50–60%
Negative anti-CCP (unless RA present)
Eye tests
Dry Schirmer's tests
Positive fluorescent dye tests
Histology
Minor salivary glands: Lymphocyte infiltration

Table 12.1 The main diagnostic features of Sjögren's syndrome. A list of diagnostic features in Sjögren's syndrome. ANA, antinuclear antibodies; anti-CCP, anti-citrullinated peptides; CRP, C-reactive protein; ESR, erythrocyte sedimentation rate.

The test is crude (by ophthalmological standards) and formal ophthalmological assessment, including a dry eye test such as Rose bengal staining, is also advised. Rose bengal is a dye which, when dropped on to the cornea, stains devitalised or damaged epithelium in the conjunctiva (Figure 12.7). Examination shows the roughened or punctate pattern of keratitis.

Immunology

The infiltration of salivary glands is predominantly lymphocytic, and involves CD4+ T-helper/memory cells. Early on, the infiltrate is around the ducts, and later replaces the functional tissue.

Although a variety of auto-antibodies – ANA, anti-thyroid, celiac antibodies, rheumatoid factors – are produced, the predominant and most specific antibodies are those directed against Ro and La antibodies.

Ro (also known as SSA) is primarily localised in the cytoplasm and thus, in some cases, conventional anti-nuclear staining may remain negative. Anti-Ro antibodies are found more frequently in patients with earlier disease onset, longer duration, prominent parotid enlargement, and more intense infiltration of the salivary glands.

Furthermore, anti-Ro and anti-La antibodies correlate with other disease manifestations such as purpura, leukopenia, and polyclonal gammopathy. The association of anti-Ro antibodies with neonatal lupus and congenital heart block is discussed in Chapter 16.

Other diagnostic tests

Lip biopsy

Biopsy of a minor salivary gland (pinhead sized glands in the lip) gives, in most cases, a mirror image of the pathology taking place in the larger

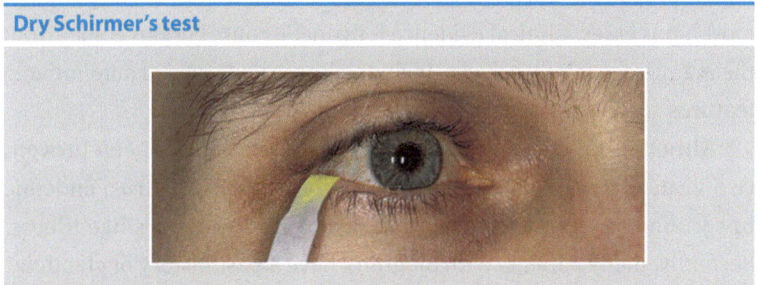

Figure 12.6 Dry Schirmer's test. The Schirmer's test is a method of measuring aqueous tear production and involves placing small strips of filter paper under the lower eyelid. Sicca syndrome in Sjögren's syndrome can be easily assessed by this test.

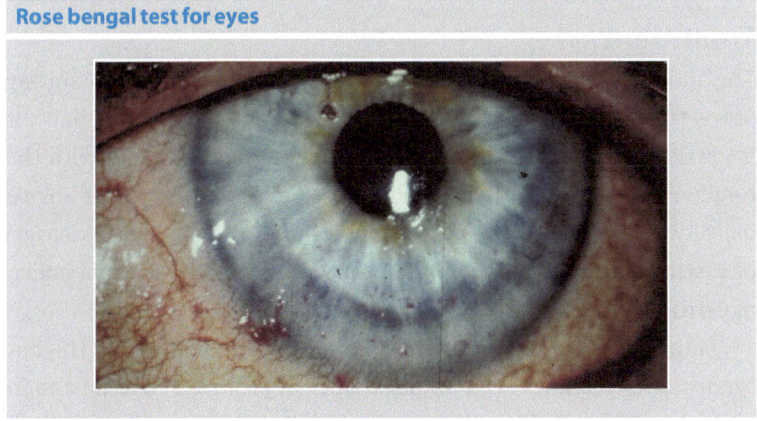

Figure 12.7 Rose bengal test for eyes. The rose bengal staining test is used patients suspected of having Sjögren's syndrome to determine the presence of keratoconjunctivitis sicca (dry eye syndrome).

glands such as the parotid. The biopsy, a small incision in the lower lip, can cause discomfort and is not routinely used.

Scintigraphy
Isotope scanning using technetium-99 measures the rate of secretion from the salivary glands into the mouth. In Sjögren's, the secretion of labelled saliva is delayed.

Etiology
As with lupus, there is evidence for genetic, environmental and hormonal factors in the pathogenesis of Sjögren's syndrome. There is a marked female preponderance, though the age of onset is much later than that of most lupus cases. Clinical evidence for genetic contributions comes from the many large family cohorts, including those with related autoimmune features such as celiac, thyroid and rheumatoid diseases.

Although no clear-cut environmental causes have been proven, two viruses have been implicated. Firstly, hepatitis C virus, endemic in certain countries such as Egypt, can cause a Sjögren's-like illness. Secondly, many patients with Sjögren's have a past history of glandular fever caused by the Epstein-Barr (E-B) virus, that is often severe and lasting many months. While the E-B virus is thus under suspicion as a cause of Sjögren's, more evidence is needed.

Treatment
The antimalarial drug hydroxychloroquine (Plaquenil) is the mainstay of treatment for Sjögren's. In doses ranging from 200–400 mg daily, it is particularly effective in improving the fatigue associated with the condition. For acute flares, short courses of steroids (5–10 mg prednisolone daily for 1–2 weeks) can be very effective. For those with more extensive or resistant disease, azathioprine (and more recently mycophenolate mofetil) is widely used.

Many patients with Sjögren's syndrome suffer features of Hughes syndrome (sometimes even in the absence of positive aPL tests) and in such cases, the addition of low dose aspirin is helpful.

Chapter 13

Hughes syndrome
(the antiphospholipid syndrome)

An increasingly important link between aPL antibodies and a clinical syndrome is becoming recognized worldwide. This syndrome, known as the antiphospholipid syndrome (APS) or Hughes syndrome, is a prothrombotic disorder leading to both arterial and venous thrombosis and, in pregnancy, recurrent abortion and pregnancy loss (Figure 13.1).

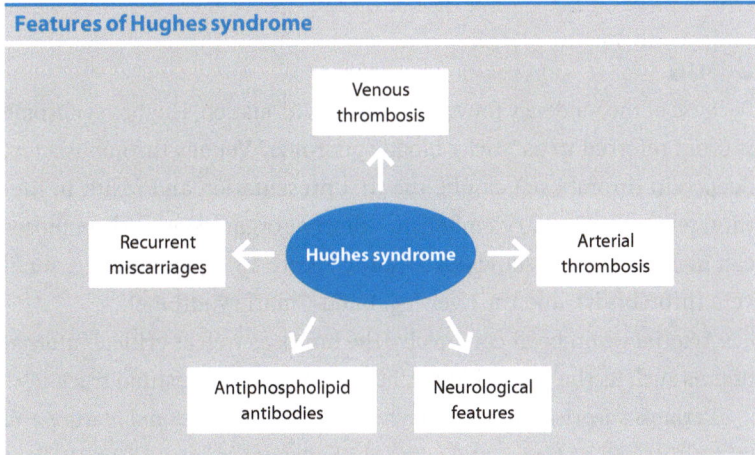

Features of Hughes syndrome

Figure 13.1 Features of Hughes syndrome. A diagram detailing the major features of Hughes syndrome, including thrombosis, presence of antiphospholipid antibodies and recurrent miscarriage.

Introduction

The Wassermann reaction (WR), an early test for syphilis, is essentially the forerunner of the modern aPL test. For over half a century, it was recognized that a "false-positive WR" could be found in some patients with lupus.

In 1983, we described the clinical details of a syndrome characterised by recurrent thrombosis, neurological disease, occasional thrombocyto-penia, and recurrent pregnancy loss. Critically, the thromboses involved arteries (eg, stroke and heart attack) as well as veins.

We identified the link with aPL antibodies and set up sensitive assays for their detection. We also recognized that the syndrome could exist outside of lupus and called the syndrome the antiphospholipid syndrome (APS). Technically, the antibodies aren't specifically directed to phospho-lipids, but protein co-factors such as prothrombin and beta 2 glycoprotein 1 are required for the pathological clotting process to go ahead. For this reason, the alternative, simpler title "Hughes syndrome" was proposed by the international APS congress in 1992. The main clinical criteria for Hughes syndrome are listed in Table 13.1.

Blood

Because of the tendency toward thrombosis formation, Hughes syndrome is often referred to as 'sticky blood syndrome.' Venous thrombosis (eg, deep vein thrombosis) can be the first presentation and result in life-threatening pulmonary embolism. Internal organ venous thromboses can include adrenal glands (Addison's; Figure 13.2), kidneys (eg, renal vein thrombosis), and the liver (eg, Budd-Chiari syndrome).

Arterial thrombosis can involve the limbs, as well as critical internal organs such as the brain, kidney, heart, and gastrointestinal tract.

Perhaps surprisingly, thrombocytopenia is an occasional feature and sometimes can be severe and acute, with platelet counts of 10×10^9/L or less but more commonly with borderline counts of 100×10^9 to 120×10^9/L.

Pregnancy

There is an increased risk of miscarriage and fetal death that is pre-dominantly due to placental ischemia. In fact, Hughes syndrome is now

Main criteria for Hughes syndrome

1. Venous thrombosis

- Deep vein thrombosis (DVT)
- Pulmonary embolism
- Renal vein thrombosis
- Saggital sinus thrombosis

2. Arterial thrombosis

- Stroke
- Renal artery thrombosis
- Myocardial infarction
- Bowel ischemia

Organs:
- Brain
- Eye
- Kidney
- Liver
- Adrenal glands

3. Pregnancy loss

- Multiple miscarriages
- Late fetal loss
- Intra uterine growth retardation
- Infertility (some cases)

4. Wide variety of neurological features

- Epilepsy
- Memory loss
- Movement disorder

5. Occasional thrombocytopenia

Table 13.1 Main criteria for Hughes syndrome. A list of the main criteria used to diagnose Hughes syndrome.

Adrenal infarction in Hughes syndrome

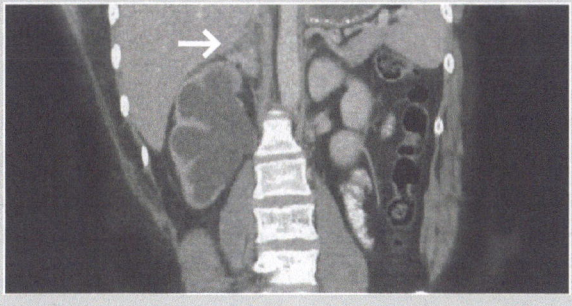

Figure 13.2 Adrenal infarction in Hughes syndrome. Adrenal infarction (arrowed) due to thrombosis in the adrenal glands. Infarction is more common in patients with Hughes syndrome.

recognized as the most common treatable cause of recurrent miscarriage and some women can suffer a dozen or more miscarriages without treatment. Late pregnancy loss, as well as other late pregnancy complications, is common. However, treatment has revolutionised the outcome for these women and is one of the success stories of modern medicine.

Brain

Brain involvement is a prominent feature and signs and symptoms cover the whole spectrum of neurology. The brain is peculiarly sensitive to the hypoxia associated with the 'blood sludging' effect of Hughes syndrome. The two most common features are migraine (often going back to childhood) and memory loss, causing patients to frequently express concern about Alzheimer's disease. Strokes in patients with Hughes syndrome account for up to one in five young strokes (aged under 45) and can recur if untreated.

Other neurological presentations include epilepsy (up to one in five of idiopathic teenage epilepsy cases tested aPL-positive), visual disturbance, balance problems and transverse myelopathy. Some cases have proved to be indistinguishable from multiple sclerosis. Chorea and movement disorders are also seen.

Heart

Heart valve thrombosis and damage (eg, Libman-Sacks endocarditis) are well documented (Figure 13.3). Myocardial ischemia and heart attack are also seen. Recent studies have suggested that Hughes syndrome might prove to be a significant cause of heart attack in younger patients.

Other organs

Skin ischemia and skin ulceration is often seen. A very common feature is livedo reticularis (see Chapter 3), a clinical finding which appears to be a very significant pointer towards thrombosis in Hughes syndrome.

Lung involvement can range from acute (pulmonary embolism; Figure 13.4) to insidious (pulmonary hypertension).

In the kidney, small vessel thrombosis can be a significant factor in the pathology in patients with lupus who are aPL-positive.

Cardiac valve deformity in Hughes syndrome

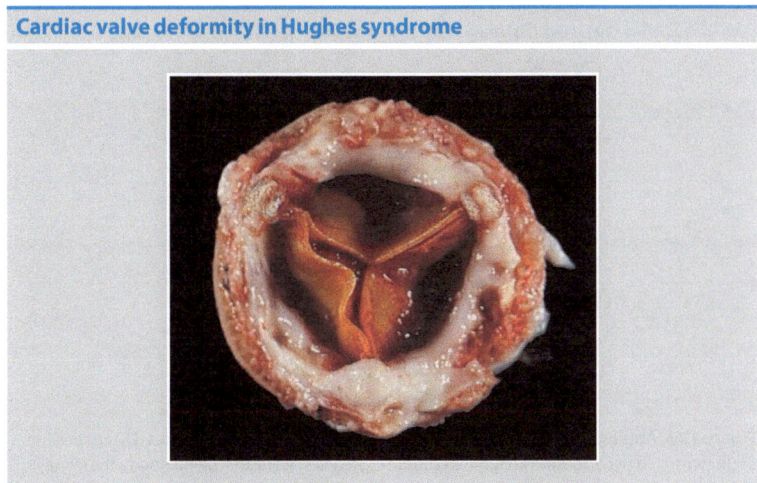

Figure 13.3 Cardiac valve deformity in Hughes syndrome. An estimated 30% of patients with Hughes syndrome have valvular lesions.

Pulmonary embolism in Hughes syndrome

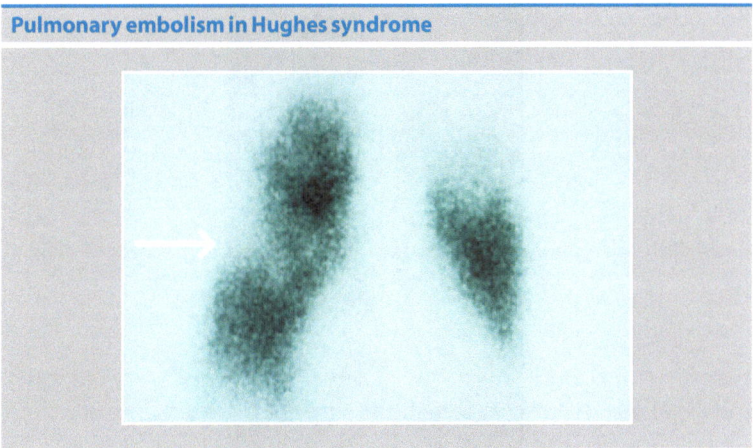

Figure 13.4 Pulmonary embolism in Hughes syndrome. Mismatched ventilation perfusion scan showing pulmonary embolism in Hughes syndrome.

Renal artery thrombosis results from a focal narrowing of an otherwise healthy looking renal artery, leading to hypertension (Figure 13.5). Similar focal occlusions are seen in other arteries such as the carotid and the celiac (Figure 13.6) and mesenteric arteries (the latter leading to mesenteric angina).

Angiogram showing renal artery stenosis in Hughes syndrome

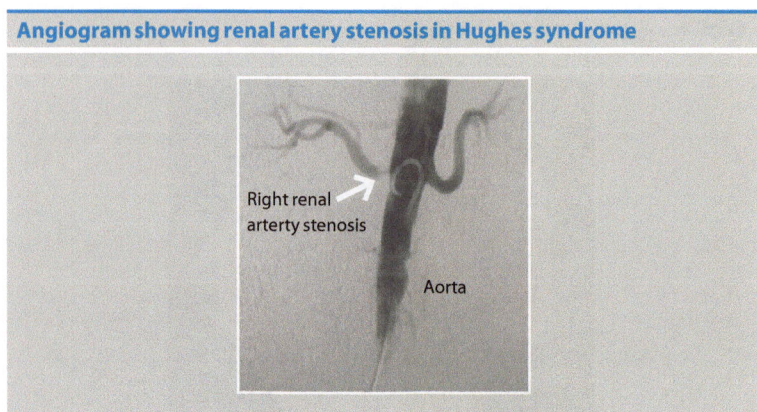

Figure 13.5 Angiogram showing renal artery stenosis in Hughes syndrome. Often presents as uncontrolled hypertension in Hughes syndrome. Stenosis can restrict blood flow to the kidney, impairing function.

Celiac artery thrombosis in Hughes syndrome

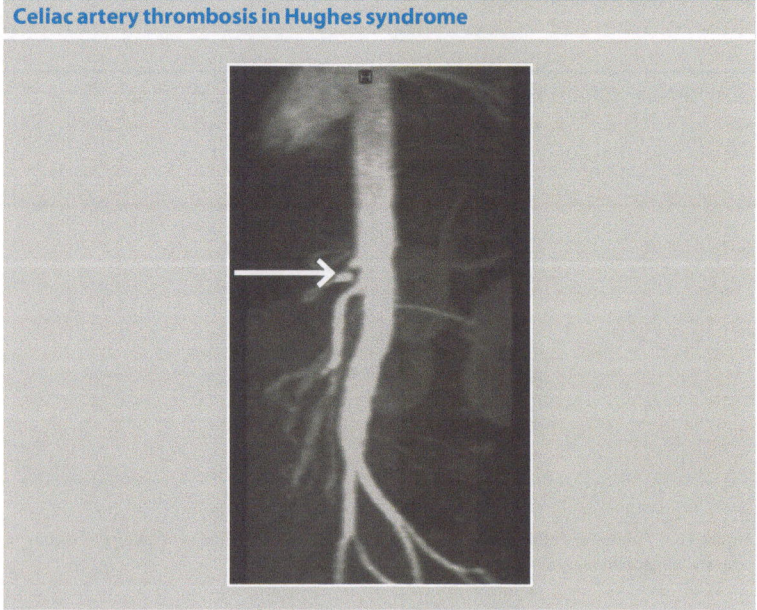

Figure 13.6 Celiac artery thrombosis in Hughes syndrome. Thrombosis is clearly visible on the celiac trunk (see arrow).

In the locomotor system, focal ischemia can lead to bone fracture (especially in the metatarsals; Figure 13.7) and joint ischemia (eg, avascular necrosis of the head of the femur).

Main criteria for Hughes syndrome

1. Venous thrombosis

- Deep vein thrombosis (DVT)
- Pulmonary embolism
- Renal vein thrombosis
- Saggital sinus thrombosis

2. Arterial thrombosis

- Stroke
- Renal artery thrombosis
- Myocardial infarction
- Bowel ischemia

Organs:
- Brain
- Eye
- Kidney
- Liver
- Adrenal glands

3. Pregnancy loss

- Multiple miscarriages
- Late fetal loss
- Intra uterine growth retardation
- Infertility (some cases)

4. Wide variety of neurological features

- Epilepsy
- Memory loss
- Movement disorder

5. Occasional thrombocytopenia

Table 13.1 Main criteria for Hughes syndrome. A list of the main criteria used to diagnose Hughes syndrome.

Adrenal infarction in Hughes syndrome

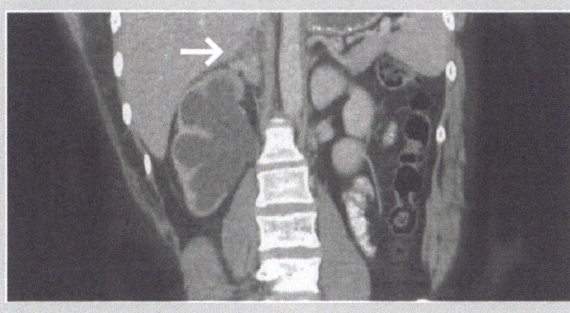

Figure 13.2 Adrenal infarction in Hughes syndrome. Adrenal infarction (arrowed) due to thrombosis in the adrenal glands. Infarction is more common in patients with Hughes syndrome.

The future

Newer anticoagulants, such as dabigatran (Pradaxa) will certainly be a welcome addition to the therapeutic armoury. So too will newer selective immunosuppressives such as the anti-B cell agents rituximab and belimumab. Anecdotally, these agents are already being tried in some more severe and resistant cases.

The description of Hughes syndrome has linked many specialities, and added a new line of diagnoses and treatment to a wide variety of common clinical conditions, ranging through balance problems, to miscarriages, to epilepsy, to migraine, to heart attack. With so many disciplines involved, spreading the word to busy clinicians is a priority.

Chapter 14

Mixed connective tissue disease (and overlap syndromes)

In 1966, Dr Gordon Sharp described a condition characterised by Raynaud's, joint problems, 'overlapping' features of lupus and scleroderma and defined by the presence of a specific antibody: anti-ribonucleoprotein (anti-RNP). Although initially criticized as a concept, the condition he described, mixed connective tissue disease (MCTD), has been accepted by the medical community and is often referred to as Sharp's disease. Indeed with its link to a single antibody that is often in high titer, it is one of the most intriguing of the connective tissue diseases.

Clinical features

Raynaud's phenomenon

With the possible exception of scleroderma, no other condition displays such severe Raynaud's syndrome. The classic triad of white, blue and red skin discoloration can affect both toes and fingers, even sometimes bizarrely just a single digit. The ischemia can be severe, leading to ulceration and even loss of one or more digits (Figure 14.1).

Joints and tendons

A common and notable feature is of 'sausage-like' swelling of fingers. Due to a combination of tendonitis and subcutaneous swelling, this often leads to marked stiffness and puffiness of the fingers. There may

Raynaud's phenomenon

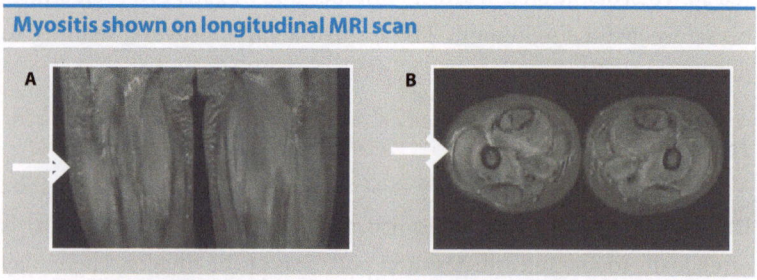

Figure 14.1 Raynaud's phenomenon. Discoloration of the digits due to restricted blood supply. Raynaud's phenomeron can also cause numbness and pain.

be tendon crepitus and other tendons in the shoulder or lower limbs, for example, can be affected.

Joint swelling in most cases is mild, though a sub-group of patients do develop rheumatoid-like disease, reinforcing the concept of 'mixed' connective tissue disease.

Muscles

In some cases, a true inflammatory myopathy occurs, with muscle weakness, raised creatine phosphokinase and abnormal electromyogram. Indeed myositis can be the predominant and presenting feature (Figure 14.2A and B). Anti-RNP measurement is an important part of the workup of cases of myositis.

Myositis shown on longitudinal MRI scan

A B

Figure 14.2A and B Myositis shown on transverse MRI scan. A Longitudinal MRI scan. **B** Transverse MRI scan. Bright areas indicate inflamed muscles, usually associated with elevated creatine kinase.

Other organs

As with other causes of Raynaud's, esophageal problems can be severe. These include dysphagia, reflux, and even stenosis. Systemic features can mimic lupus, with photosensitivity, pleurisy, and pericarditis. Severe renal involvement in MCTD is rare.

Immunology

One of the interesting features of MCTD is its immunological profile. Unlike lupus, which is characterised by a veritable rainbow of antibodies (over 100 have been described), MCTD is essentially characterised by one antibody: anti-RNP. In ANA testing, this shows up as a 'speckled' pattern that is often present in high titers, even at a dilution of over one in a million.

As well as this extraordinarily high titer of anti-RNP in some patients, other fairly nonspecific signs of immunological over-activity include raised gammaglobulin levels and (occasionally) a positive rheumatoid factor test.

Outcome

MCTD has been almost universally regarded as an overlap of Sjörgren's syndrome, scleroderma, Raynaud's, myositis and rheumatoid arthritis but generally with a more benign outcome (Figure 14.3). While this may be true for overall prognosis, in clinical practice, MCTD is often more

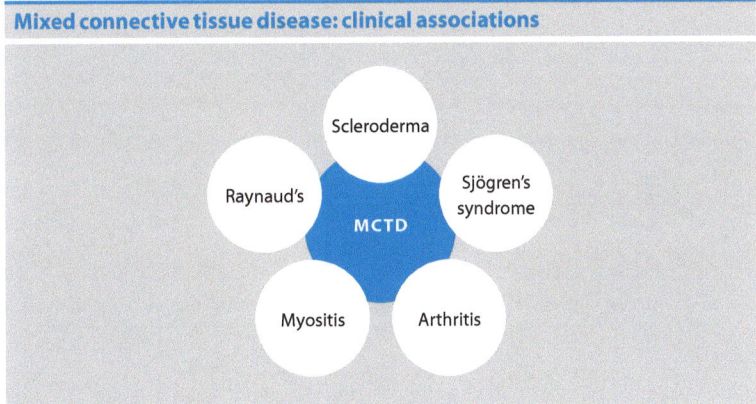

Figure 14.3 Mixed connective tissue disease: clinical associations. An overlap of scleroderma, myositis, Sjögren's syndrome, arthritis, and Raynaud's phenomenon.

troublesome and more resistant to management than any of its better known relatives.

In many patients moderately high steroid doses (eg, 20 mg daily) are needed to control symptoms, while in others, particularly those with prominent muscle or joint involvement, are given steroid sparing agents such as methotrexate or anti-tumor necrosis factor (TNF) agents.

Chapter 15

Vasculitis

Although much of the pathology of lupus is in fact small vessel vasculitis, it is customary to separate the group of disorders grouped under the 'primary' vasculitis label.

The group differs from lupus in a number of ways including the relatively few immunological markers (anti-neutrophil cytoplasmic antibodies being an exception), and the high inflammatory markers such as ESR, CRP, leukocyte count and (often) high platelet counts.

Classification

There have been many attempts to classify this heterogeneous group of diseases. By far the simplest and most practical for the clinician is by vessel size (Figure 15.1). Thus Takayasu's arteritis affects large (and very large) arteries such as the aorta; polyarteritis nodosa and Wegener's granulomatosis affects smaller arteries; a variety of inflammatory arteritides (eg, allergic vasculitis) affect the smallest vessels.

For the clinician, these diseases are generally clearly distinguishable from lupus. A few of the major vasculitides are discussed briefly here.

Wegener's granulomatosis

This once uniformly fatal disease is now largely treatable with cyclophosphamide.

Classification of vasculitis

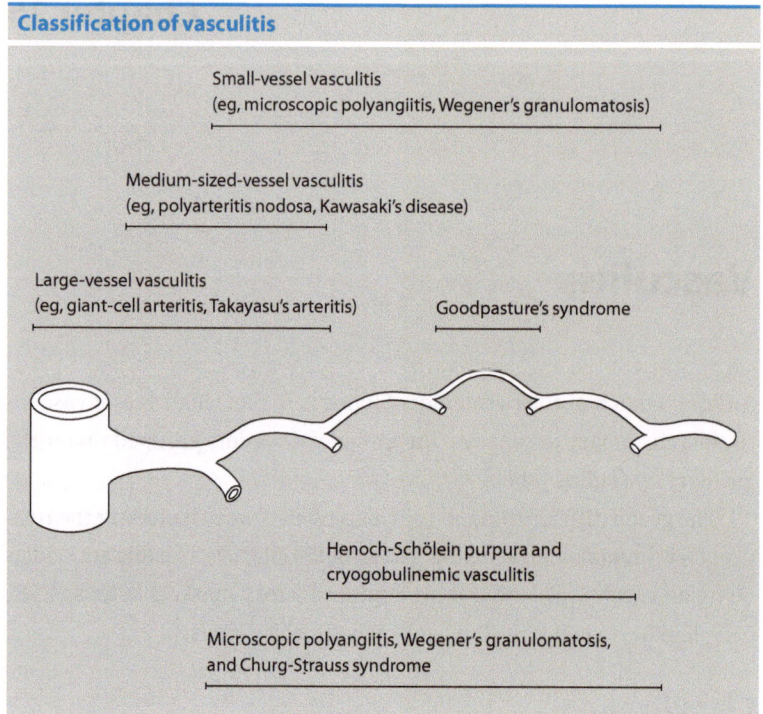

Small-vessel vasculitis
(eg, microscopic polyangiitis, Wegener's granulomatosis)

Medium-sized-vessel vasculitis
(eg, polyarteritis nodosa, Kawasaki's disease)

Large-vessel vasculitis
(eg, giant-cell arteritis, Takayasu's arteritis)

Goodpasture's syndrome

Henoch-Schölein purpura and
cryogobulinemic vasculitis

Microscopic polyangiitis, Wegener's granulomatosis,
and Churg-Strauss syndrome

Figure 15.1 Classification of vasculitis. Vasculitis indicates inflammation of blood vessels. Classification is primarily based on blood vessel size.

The condition consists of two features: granulomatous necrosis, affecting sinuses and lungs, and more widespread inflammatory vasculitis, affecting the arteries of limbs as well as internal organs.

The classical picture is development of chronic sinusitis, leading to blood-stained and necrotic nasal discharge. CT scans of the sinuses show filling of the sinuses and (later) erosion of bone (Figure 15.2). Granulomatous lesions can fill the eye socket leading to exophthalmos (Figure 15.3). The lungs are commonly involved, with almost the full spectrum of pulmonary presentations ranging from pleural effusions to 'cannonball' lung pictures (Figure 15.4). Features of Wegener's granulomatosis also include peripheral neuropathy (including mononeuritis multiplex), vasculitic skin lesions (Figure 15.5), liver and kidney involvement (Figure 15.6) and myocardial infarction.

Wegener's granulomatosis – CT scan of sinus showing collapsed nasal bridge

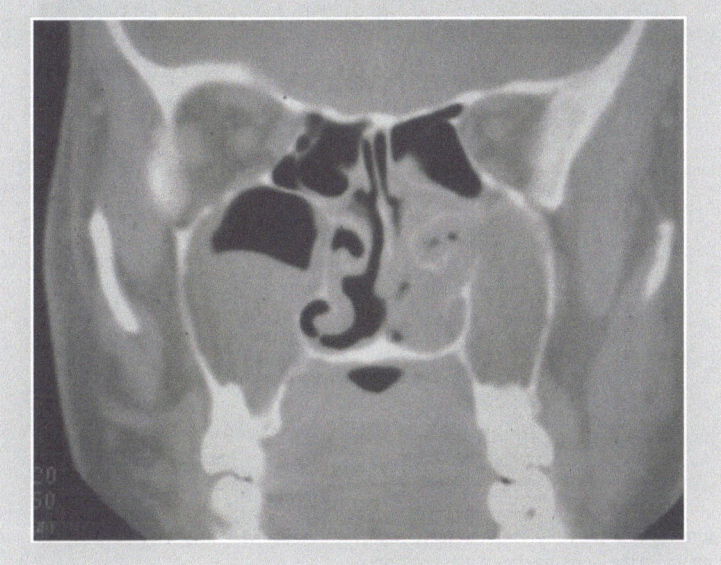

Figure 15.2 Wegener's granulomatosis – CT scan of sinus showing collapsed nasal septum. Wegener's granulomatosis can cause bony erosions, destruction and mucosal thickening.

Intra-orbital mass in Wegener's granulomatosis

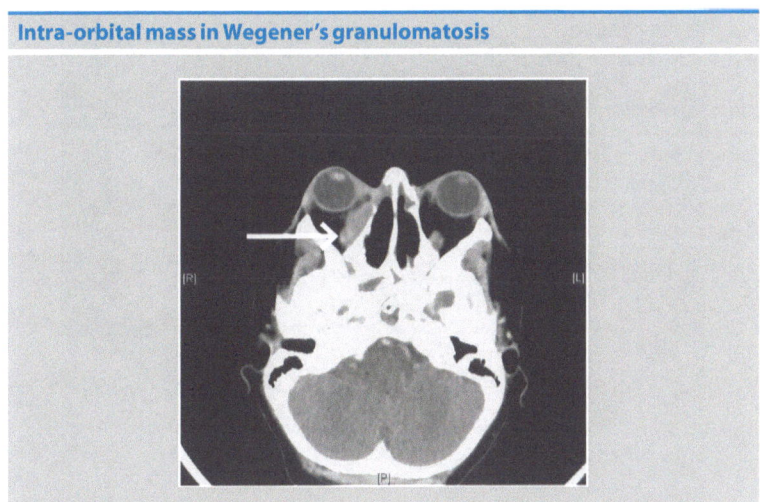

Figure 15.3 Intra-orbital mass in Wegener's granulomatosis. An intra-orbital granuloma (arrowed) in Wegener's granulomatosis can affect vision and, in severe cases, destroy the orbit.

Wegener's granulomatosis – lung involvement

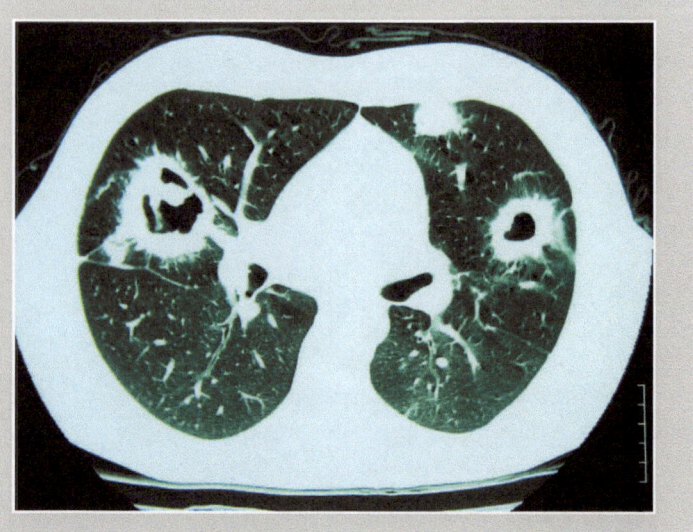

Figure 15.4 Wegener's granulomatosis – lung involvement. Lung nodules and cavity formation in the lungs may present as hemoptysis.

Wegener's granulomatosis – skin ulcers

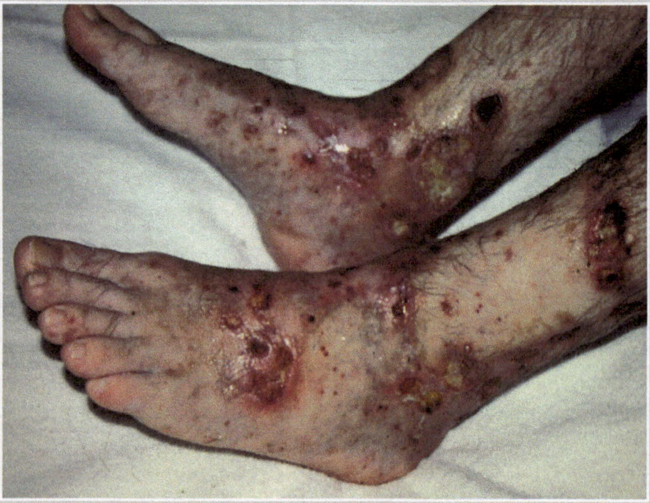

Figure 15.5 Wegener's granulomatosis – skin ulcers. Severe cutaneous ulcers in a patient with Wegener's granulomatosis.

Renal involvement in Wegener's granulomatosis

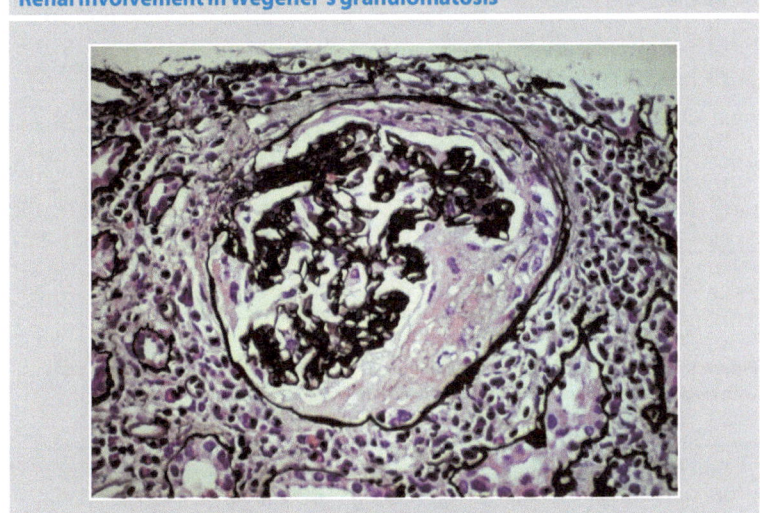

Figure 15.6 Renal involvement in Wegener's granulomatosis. Necrotising glomerulonephritis, showing necrotic glomerulus scarring and inflammatory infiltrate.

Diagnosis

The clinical picture of vasculitis is usually well defined and diagnosis is generally straightforward.

Inflammatory features include a raised CRP (often very high), raised WBC (sometimes over 20 x 10^9/L and high platelets (often over 400 x 10^9/L).

CT scans of sinuses and chest X-rays may show the characteristic pictures. The ultimate proof of the diagnosis comes from tissue biopsy (eg, bronchoscopy), though obtaining clear histological proof in a newly sick patient with Wegener's granulomatosis is the exception rather than the rule.

The one immunologically useful test is anti-neutrophil cytoplasmic antibody (ANCA). It was found some years ago that most patients with Wegener's granulomatosis had a circulating antibody directed against a constituent of cytoplasm. Two main antigens have since been recognized: myeloperoxidase, now known to be responsible for the P-ANCA antibodies. C-ANCA (an easy memo is 'C for classical' as in classical Wegener's) is the specific test for Wegener's granulomatosis (Figure 15.7A). P-ANCA, by contrast, is seen in a number of inflammatory diseases (Figure 15.7B).

C-ANCA

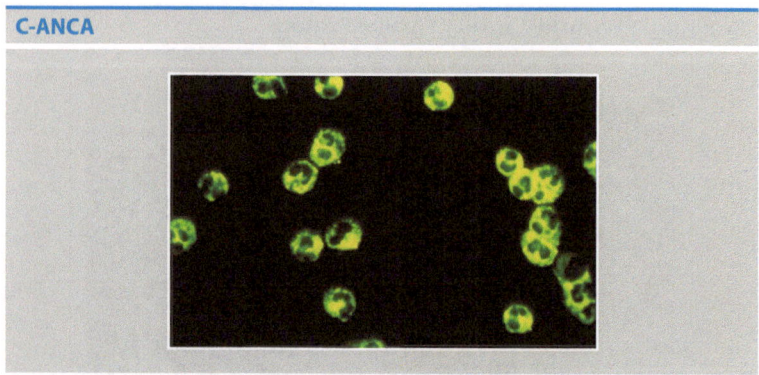

Figure 15.7A C-ANCA. Anti cytoplasmic antibodies (PR3) are seen in more than 70% of patients with Wegener's granulomatosis. ANCA, antineutrophil cystoplasmic antibodies.

P-ANCA

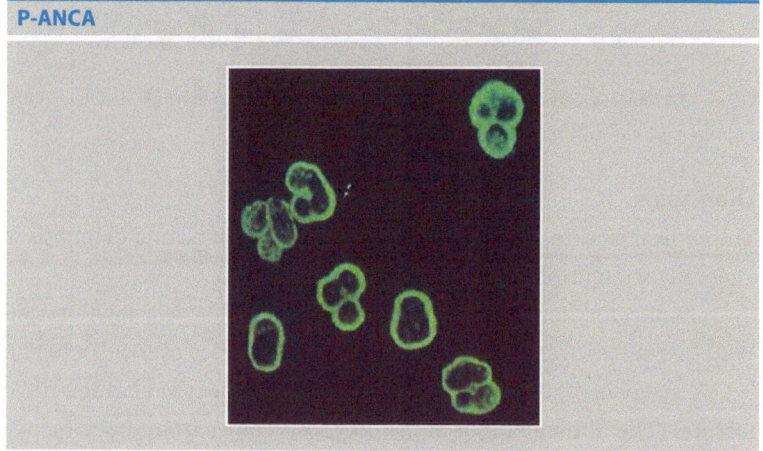

Figure 15.7B P-ANCA. Anti cytoplasmic antibodies (myeloperoxidase) are seen in various types of vasculitis including Wegener's granulomatosis, Churg-Strauss syndrome and polyarteritis nodosa. ANCA, antineutrophil cytoplasmic antibodies.

Treatment

The use of pulse cyclophosphamide has revolutionised the treatment of Wegener's granulomatosis. Eye swelling, sinus obstruction, and lung shadows often melt dramatically following even the first IV pulse of the drug. Thus, speedy diagnosis is vital.

Most Wegener's granulomatosis patients treated with IV cyclophosphamide attain remission, though life-long observation is mandatory, as the disease can frequently flare.

Polyarteritis nodosa

Polyarteritis nodosa (PAN) is a rarely seen extreme form of vasculitis, often presenting dramatically, with a high early fatality rate. The pathological picture is one of inflammation affecting mainly medium-sized arteries that is often so intense that it casues weaknesses in the vessel wall and secondary aneurysm formation, resulting in the knotted ('nodosa') formation which gives the disease its name.

The clinical picture is one of extreme and acute inflammatory disease, including nephritis, hypertension, lung lesions, myocardial infarction, gut necrosis (Figure 15.8), testicular infarction (Figure 15.9) and mononeuritis multiplex, a nervous system disorder that involves pathognomonic 'picking off' of peripheral nerves, often in a seemingly random pattern.

Peripheral white blood counts can exceed 30 x 10^9/L, and C-reactive protein values are usually over 100.

In 1970, an association between PAN and hepatitis B was identified. Subsequent series of PAN cases included many cases of drug addiction and hepatitis B infection, and serological studies demonstrated circulating immune complexes of hepatitis B virus and antibody.

As with Wegener's granulomatosis, PAN treatment is initially with a combination of steroids and immunosuppressives. Unlike Wegener's granulomatosis however, the illness is usually a 'one shot' condition: life-threatening at first but, if controlled, usually remains dormant thereafter.

Mesenteric involvement in polyarteritis nodusa

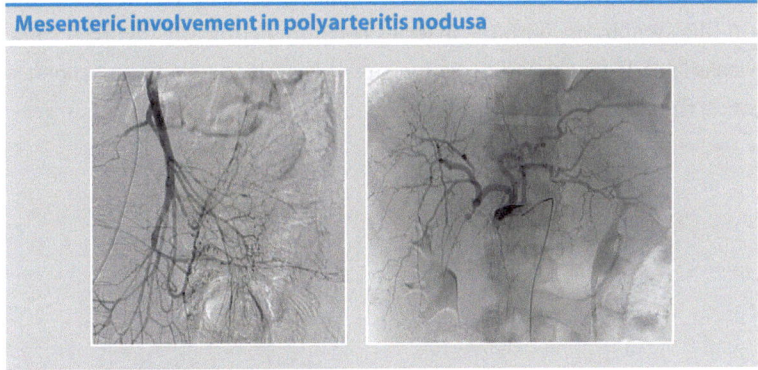

Figure 15.8 Mesenteric involvement in polyarteritis nodusa. Micro-aneurysms on mesenteric blood vessels in polyarteritis nodusa.

Testicular infarction in polyarteritis nodosa

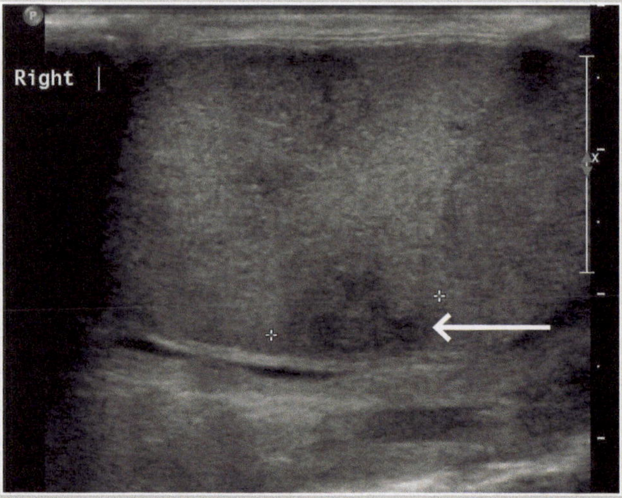

Figure 15.9 Testicular infarction in polyarteritis nodusa. An ultrasound image showing testicular infarction (dark area; arrowed) in a patient with polyarteritis nodusa. Infarction can occur if polyarteritis nodusa is severe enough to affect blood supply and cause necrosis.

Takayasu's arteritis

This acute onset vasculitis affects the aortic arch and its main branches (Figure 15.10), classically resulting in absent arm pulses (but with normal leg pulses). Cerebral and ocular circulation can be affected. The etiology is unknown but the illness is often biphasic, starting with generalised flu-like symptoms, with the arteries becoming clinically involved some weeks later. If caught early, treatment is with steroids and immunosuppressives, though the later occlusive sequelae may require vascular surgery.

Takayasu's arteritis

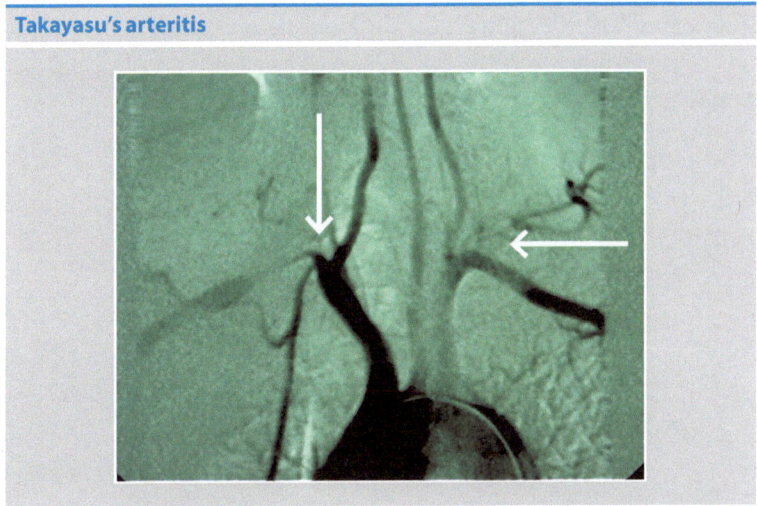

Figure 15.10 Takayasu's arteritis. Complete occlusion of right subclavian and left common carotid arties due to Takayasu's arteritis. This condition generally involves large blood vessels.

PART FIVE

Lupus-related topics

Chapter 16

Lupus-related topics

Lupus and pregnancy

Lupus used to be regarded as a contraindication to pregnancy. Sadly, many patients with lupus were strongly advised against becoming pregnant. Times have changed and indeed many lupus centres now run busy pregnancy clinics. We now recognise that lupus itself generally has no major impact on pregnancy outcome (those with marked renal impairment or hypertension excepted).

The major risk in lupus is related to aPL antibodies. As with the Hughes syndrome, patients with lupus who are aPL-positive have an increased chance not only of repeated pregnancy loss, but also of other pregnancy related conditions, notably intrauterine growth retardation. Thus, aPL-positive patients with lupus need to be considered for aspirin and/or heparin treatment during pregnancy.

Patients with lupus carrying anti-Ro antibodies are at risk of giving birth to an infant with congenital heart block, a rare development which occurs in 1 in 500 births (Figure 16.1). There is a very low risk, but the risk increases to 1 in 20 in pregnancies following a first child born with a congenital heart block.

Lupus in children

Although lupus normally affects individuals in their teens and upwards (in girls after the start of menstruation), lupus can and does affect children (and even toddlers).

An ECG showing complete heart block

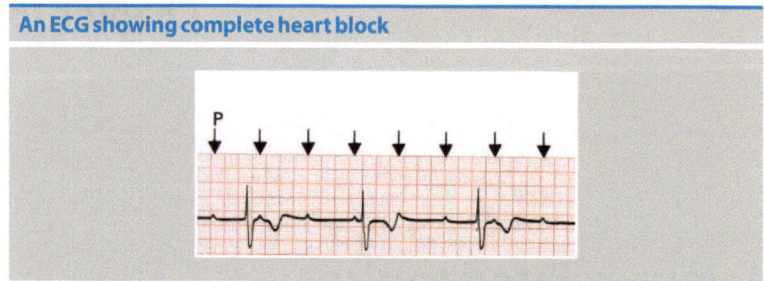

Figure 16.1 An ECG showing complete heart block. An ECG showing P Wave (arrows) and QRS complexes occuring independently. Congenital heart block is a rare complication seen in newborns due to transplacental transfer of Ro antibodies from the mother.

The clinical patterns in children are similar to those in adults, and in general, treatment options are the same. Provided the diagnosis is made quickly and treatment is started immediately, the prognosis is no worse than that in adults. In our practice, we have dozens of patients in whom lupus first presented under the age of 12 but are now in remission and no longer taking strong medicines.

Lupus and late arterial disease

In recent years, it has been recognized that patients with lupus have an increased risk of atheromatous disease later in life (in the 40s, 50s and 60s), including coronary disease and stroke; so much so that lupus has been labelled by some 'the new diabetes'. The cause(s) of this phenomenon are not yet clear, but possible contributors include steroids, chronic inflammation, and renal disease.

Lupus and malignancy

Despite many patients with lupus receiving immune-altering drugs, coming in and out of hospitals and presumably coming into contact with a multitude of viruses, malignancy in lupus is strikingly uncommon.

However, one clinical association may have influenced publications in the past: Non-Hodgkin's lymphoma (NHL) has an increased prevalence in Sjögren's patients, notably those patients with enlarged parotids and other glands. This group of patients is older than the average lupus age (often in their 60s) and immunologically different (for instance, anti-dsDNA negative). However, it is possible that some previous studies claiming a higher NHL risk in lupus may well have included patients from the Sjögren's group, as the average age in some reported series strongly suggests this.

A second caveat concerns cervical cancer. Many years ago it was reported that many patients with lupus had abnormal cervical smears. We wondered whether either the vaginal dryness or perhaps the medication they were prescribed was the underlying reason. Almost universally, these abnormal smears turned out to be benign and cervical cancer has not been an increased problem in our patients.

Drug-induced lupus

Other factors reported as triggering lupus are drugs, including hydralazine (a blood pressure drug), Septrin, (an older sulphur-containing antibiotic), and anti-TNF drugs (used for rheumatoid arthritis) (Figure 16.2).

In some of these examples, the condition usually known as drug-induced lupus, rarely progresses to kidney disease and usually (with the exception of Septrin) disappears on stopping the offending drug.

One notable cause of drug-induced lupus is minocycline, an antibiotic that has been widely used for the treatment of acne in teenagers. In a small number, the recipient developed joint pains and other features of

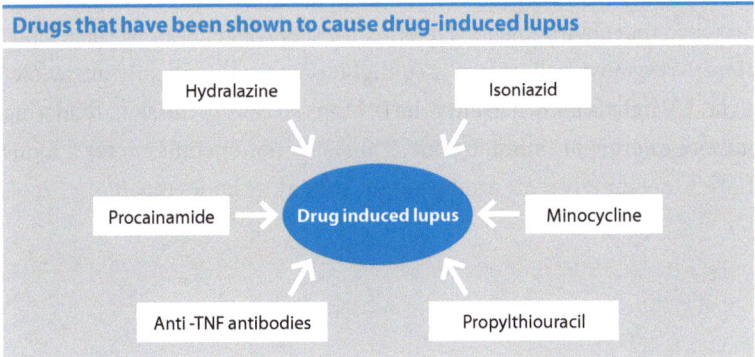

Figure 16.2 Drugs that have been shown to cause drug-induced lupus. A number of drugs may produce a lupus-like syndrome. The adverse effects generally clear up upon stopping the offending treatment.

lupus. Perhaps, not surprisingly, the connection in some cases was not made and the drug-induced lupus became severe.

Flares of lupus have also been occasionally reported after vaccination and immunization, and suggestions have been made that some solvents or adjuvants used in vaccines may have had a triggering effect. However, one of the most common triggers of lupus appears to be stress. The mechanisms are probably complex. There is plenty of evidence, for example, that stress has measurable effects on the immune system. Clinically, some cases dramatically highlight the link. For example, one of our patients suffered two family bereavements in a year and in both cases, these events were followed by a severe drop in platelet counts. Coincidence perhaps, but there are numerous such cases in any large lupus practice.

Lupus: soil versus seed

Clearly, lupus has something of a genetic basis, as there are many families with more than one lupus sufferer. Twin studies show an increased lupus risk in the twin sibling of a patient with lupus. Furthermore, relatives of lupus patients have an increased propensity to other auto-immune conditions such as thyroid disease, Sjögren's and rheumatoid arthritis.

Studies by genetic departments are, not surprisingly, confirming these observations and in time, it may be possible to find a genetic 'fingerprint' for lupus (see Figure 2.4). As well as genetic factors, it is increasingly accepted that environmental factors can either trigger or exacerbate lupus flares. The most well known is sunlight, or more specifically ultraviolet light. UV light is known to alter the DNA in the cells of the skin, rendering it more allergic or immunogenic. Thus, it is not uncommon for a lupus flare to seemingly start after a sunny holiday or honeymoon.